Gut Health Simple

An Empowering Guide to Achieving Optimal Health and Vitality Through Nourishing Your Gut

Claudia Miller

© **Copyright 2022 - All rights reserved.**

The content contained within this book may not be reproduced, duplicated or transmitted without direct written permission from the author or the publisher.

Under no circumstances will any blame or legal responsibility be held against the publisher, or author, for any damages, reparation, or monetary loss due to the information contained within this book, either directly or indirectly.

Legal Notice:

This book is copyright protected. It is only for personal use. You cannot amend, distribute, sell, use, quote or paraphrase any part, or the content within this book, without the consent of the author or publisher.

Disclaimer Notice:

Please note the information contained within this document is for educational and entertainment purposes only. All effort has been executed to present accurate, up to date, reliable, complete information. No warranties of any kind are declared or implied. Readers acknowledge that the author is not engaged in the rendering of legal, financial, medical or professional advice. The content within this book has been derived from various sources. Please consult a licensed professional before attempting any techniques outlined in this book.

By reading this document, the reader agrees that under no circumstances is the author responsible for any losses, direct or indirect, that are incurred as a result of the use of the information contained within this document, including, but not limited to, errors, omissions, or inaccuracies.

Table of Contents

INTRODUCTION 1
   Is it Time to Consider Taking Care of My Gut? 2

CHAPTER 1: MEET YOUR GUT 5
   SAY 'HELLO' TO YOUR GUT 6
      Your Gut Unrolled 7
      Signs Your Upper Digestive Tract is Not Okay 11
      What Can You Do to Ensure Optimal Health of Your Upper GI? 13
      Maintaining the Health of Your Lower-Digestive System—Home to Your Microbiota 18
      Identifying Problems With Your Lower-Digestive System 20
      Maintain the Health of Your Gut Bacteria 21

CHAPTER 2: A CLOSER LOOK AT YOUR GUT MICROBIOME 25
   WHAT IS YOUR GUT MICROBIOME? 25
      What Makes Your Gut Bacteria Unique? 26
      How Is Your Gut Microbiome Determined? 28
   MAINTAINING THE HEALTH OF YOUR GUT MICROBIOME 29
      Dysbiosis 30
      How to Identify Dysbiosis 33
      Dysbiosis and Leaky Gut Syndrome 35
      The Food You Eat Has a Major Impact on Your Gut Microbiome .. 40
      How to Improve Your Gut Bacteria Through Food 41
   HOW TO KNOW YOUR GUT IS HEALTHY 43
      1.   *Learn to Read Your Poop* 43
      2.   *Bloating and Gas—When Is it Okay to Fart?* 49
      3.   *Eat to Please Your Gut Bacteria* 52
   PROBLEMS WITH YOUR GUT 53
      What Is an Unhealthy Gut? 54
      A Look at Common Digestive Syndromes Related to Dysbiosis 63
   HOW DOES YOUR GUT INFLUENCE YOUR WEIGHT? 69
      Role of Gut Bacteria and Digestion for Weight Management 69
      Gut Bacteria, Hormone Management, and Weight Gain 70

CHAPTER 3: YOU AND YOUR GUT—A UNIQUE RELATIONSHIP 73

- Are You Listening to Your Gut? 74
  - Assessing the Health of Your Gut 76
- Start Journaling Your Gut Changes 79
  - Food Journal 81
  - Try the Elimination Diet Technique to Identify Food Intolerances. 84
  - Maintaining a Poop Journal—What Must You Include 93
  - The Transit Time Test 96
  - How Can I Test My Transit Time? 97
  - The Aim For 30 Test 99
  - Tips to Easily Include Plant Foods in Your Diet 103
  - Star Ingredients That are Very Gut-Friendly 106

CHAPTER 4: NOURISH YOUR BODY 109

- Factors You Can Change Easily for a Happy Gut 109
  - Start Fresh—Change the Way You Eat 110
  - Eat in Line With Your Biochemical Makeup 111
  - Balancing Blood Sugar Levels Through Sensible Eating 114
  - Your Food Journal Can Help You Monitor Your Diet 115
  - Clean Eating and Maintaining the 80% to 20% Eating Rule 116
  - The Benefits of Eating Whole Foods 121
  - The Importance of Proper Hydration 129

CHAPTER 5: HONOUR YOUR BODY AND MIND 131

- Practice Mindful Eating 131
  - How to Practise Mindful Eating 132
- Pay Attention to How Much You Move 133
  - Times Your Gut Health is Causing Your Energy Slump 134
  - Exercise and Enjoy Movement 135

CHAPTER 6: CREATE YOUR WHOLESOME KITCHEN 143

- How to Get Started—Creating Your Wholesome Kitchen 144
  - Putting Together a Nutrient-Dense Kitchen—What are the Staples? 144
  - What's the Deal With Organic Produce? 148

CHAPTER 7: TREAT YOUR TUMMY TO TASTY RECIPES 151

- Healthy Food Hacks 151
- Healthy Recipes 152

  Recipe No 1: Overnight Oats—Grab and Go Breakfast for Busy
  Mornings 152
  Recipe No 2: Protein Fruit Smoothie 154
  Recipe No 3: Butternut Squash and Kale Soup 155
  Recipe No 4: Burrito Bowls With Chicken 157

CONCLUSION 161

  Stay in Touch 161

REFERENCES 163

Introduction

"Trust your gut!"

You are about to find out that there is more to that old saying than is let on.

Did you ever think that looking after the health of your gut would help you to live a longer, healthier, and happier life?

Well, you can!

Let me introduce you to your gastrointestinal tract (GI). It's time you got updated on the overall influence your GI has on your health and wellbeing. I am not talking about just your physical health. Your gut is often responsible for the overall well-being of your mental and physical well-being. And if you have been suspicious for a long time of an underlying health issue that you think is connected to your digestive tract, my book *"Gut Health Pure and Simple"* will help you decide on the right course of action to take.

Even if you are not dealing with any health issues related to your gut, it's important to get updated on all the information I am about to present.

Getting updated on gut health will benefit you in several ways.

- Have you made a dietary change recently because you are becoming more aware of the importance of eating right to keep your gut healthy? Do you know how each type of food affects your gut and the gut microbiome?

Let's explore and learn about the benefits of eating the right type of food to feed the good bacteria there and encourage good digestion.

- Do you also know that there are certain types of food that get digested differently in your gut? Some will make you feel hungry a few moments after you eat; while some will keep you feeling fuller for longer, will aid weight loss, and even help you manage fasting diets successfully.

- Did you know that serotonin, your feel-good hormone, is mostly secreted in your gut, and that there is such a thing as the gut-brain axis (GBA) which has a neurological connection to how you feel, directly linking your gut to your immune system, your mental health, and overall well-being?

Is it Time to Consider Taking Care of My Gut?

While taking care of your gut must be a natural process that benefits you with overall health, there are subtle and not-so-subtle signs that indicate your gut may not be functioning at its optimal best.

- Gas, bloating, constipation, diarrhoea, chronic pain, and even a sudden craving for sugar are some of the symptoms people often face when their gut is not in optimal health. Learn about the causes and cures which are quite often quick fixes, for these conditions. Even conditions such as irritable bowel syndrome (IBS) can be successfully controlled by paying attention to your gut health.

- Have you been feeling off-balance recently in terms of physical and mental health; are you harbouring a general feeling of 'yuck' and do you feel as though everything is not quite alright?

- Are you on a constant see-saw when it comes to maintaining your health? Do you suddenly start to follow healthy-eating patterns and lifestyle choices to suddenly lose all resolve and go on a binge-eating schedule that you know is damaging but you have no self-control to stop?

These are signs you could be suffering from gut-related problems. And the simple techniques and tips I offer in my book will help you easily reset most of these problems by making subtle lifestyle changes. No drugs or tests or constant visits to the doctor's surgery, just a selection of healthy choices and everyday habits that will improve your mental and physical health.

Isn't it marvellous to realise that you can finally be in charge of your health and wellbeing?

That a few simple adjustments to your diet and lifestyle can change the overall health of your digestive tract which has a huge influence on your hormone secretion, weight management, and also mental health.

I am excited to open your mind to the concept of healing your body through your gut. Working in the health and wellness sector has helped me to learn, research, and understand a lot about the human digestive tract and its influence on our overall health.

Ever since earning a First Class Honours Bachelor of Science Degree, I have spent years studying gut health, and you know what?

I discovered that simple shifts and lifestyle changes coupled with a positive and determined mindset can work wonders toward improving one's health.

These are findings I am eager to share with you because I want you to experience the same transformation that many of the people I have advised are enjoying. I want to introduce you to a healthy new lifestyle away from the drudgery of endless visits to see your healthcare provider or enduring tests to find out why you feel the way you do, or even to finally learn the secret of natural weight loss by eating a combination of the right food to keep your gut bacteria happy.

I want you to embrace a healthy lifestyle just like me because I too benefited from the simple shifts I am about to teach you.

My days are now fulfilling and rewarding because I am more energised than before. I am healthier and happier now that the anxiety of dealing with feelings of ill-health is gone. I enjoy spending happy times with my husband and two daughters and I am better equipped to face life's challenges with optimism.

The secret to happiness starts deep within yourself and I will help you to manifest a stronger, healthier, and happier person who appreciates the gift of life.

Chapter 1:

Meet Your Gut

Every disease starts in your gut! This is a fact substantiated by Hippocrates II himself.

Let's substantiate that fact and start off by exploring exactly why your gut is the most important part of your biology.

Quite simply, your gut is your protective force field. Because your intestinal tract acts like a shield preventing toxins, you ingest, from reaching your bloodstream.

Sometimes this protective barrier can get disrupted due to various external and internal causes. This chapter will explore what they are and how you can prevent your gut from malfunctioning.

My research has shown me that every person's gut function is different and what they need to do to take care of it, varies between individuals. Therefore, let's look at simple fixes that you can make after identifying the type of gut you are dealing with, and with my help and research-backed advice, you can learn to cultivate a combination of healthy habits tailor-made to suit your needs and keep your gut healthy.

Say 'Hello' to Your Gut

Your gut or gastrointestinal tract (GI) begins at your mouth and ends at your anus. Therefore, it is basically in charge of everything that passes through your body.

Your GI is solely responsible for digesting the food you eat and for absorbing and supplying your body with all the essential nutrients it needs from the nutritious calories you consume.

Your GI tract will also metabolise carbs and sugars to convert them to blood glucose so your cells, muscles, and organs can absorb and store glucose energy. Your gut will also separate the good from the bad, thus, helping your body eliminate the waste.

I just described the basic and primary function of your gut; there are many more interconnected functions your gut performs that are essential to keep you in the best shape physically and mentally. Your gut microbiota is made up of trillions of bacteria that thrive there, some are good and some are bad; taking care of the good gut bacteria will ensure your digestive tract functions at its best.

When a baby is born, the gut, just like the brain, goes through a phase of rapid development because both the gut and brain are connected to ensure your immune system is functioning at its best while influencing the health of your endocrine system, which is the network that controls your hormone secretion. This connection is called the gut-brain axis or GBA.

- More than 70% of your immune cells are found in your gut which is why your gut health largely impacts the health of your immune system.

- Your gut is responsible for the regulation of your mood and your hunger because the gut microbiota produces over 90% of your serotonin which is a mood-regulator hormone, and influences the secretion of another called ghrelin, which controls your hunger levels.

- The gut microbiota is home to millions of nerve cells that constantly communicate with the brain, influencing the release of hormones and neurotransmitters (chemical proteins acting as messengers between your neurons (nerves) and other parts of your body). This connection influences the secretion of insulin, the regulation of blood glucose, the metabolization and absorption of glucose energy from the blood, appetite, and the storage of fat.

- This vital link between hormones, neurotransmitters, your brain, and your gut can influence your overall wellbeing by controlling so many aspects of your physical and mental health.

Considering that it plays such a primary role in managing your body's functions, it is important to ensure your gut remains healthy and happy for overall wellbeing and health.

Before we delve into that fascinating world consisting of billions of bacteria called your microbiome, the secretion of hormones, or learn more about digestive enzymes that help you have a good bowel movement, let's learn a bit more about each point in that very long tube that makes up your entire digestive tract.

Your Gut Unrolled

Your digestive system is a long tube that starts from your mouth and ends at your bottom. This tube has many twists and turns and will consist of the upper digestive system and the lower digestive system. Put together, your large and small intestines can measure close to 15ft. If you look at the image below, you will get a clearer idea of how your gut is coiled up inside you.

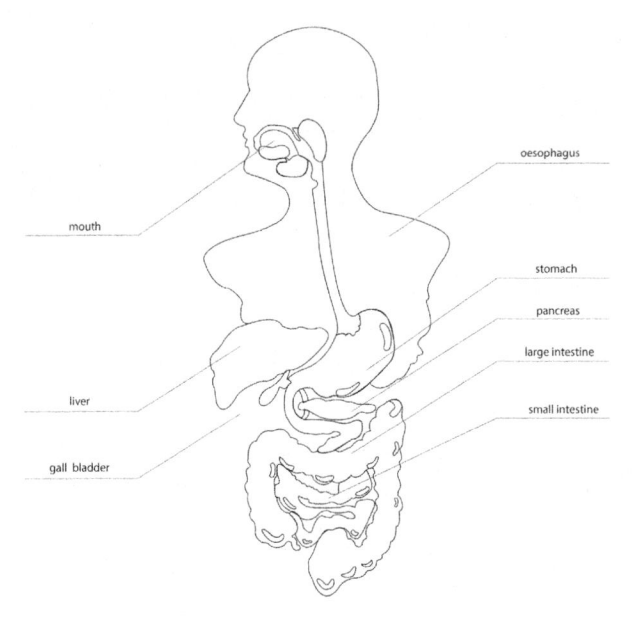

The Upper-Digestive System—Stage One

Starting from your mouth, this part of your digestive system consists of the mouth, the oesophagus, the stomach, and the starting point of the small intestines. The upper-digestive tract's main mission is to start the process of digestion by breaking down food particles so the nutrients they contain can be easily absorbed into your bloodstream.

How Does Each Part of the Upper GI Work?

- Mouth—the digestion of food starts in your mouth way before it hits the stomach. When you put food in your mouth and start to chew, your salivary glands secrete saliva, which contains enzymes that help with breaking down food particles. These enzymes first work on carbs, which means the digestion of carbs/starch begins in your mouth, which is why some cooked starches such as simple carbs make you feel hungry soon after eating them—they start to digest as soon as you pop them in your mouth.

- Oesophagus—also called the gullet, the oesophagus is a type of muscular tube through which drinks and food you chew make their way to the stomach. Food gets propelled down to the stomach through the contraction of muscles in the oesophagus.

  This muscular tube is made up of four layers:

  1. The mucosa is the lubricated outer layer that helps the food particles easily slip down the oesophagus.

  2. The submucosa that makes the mucous, helps the gullet to remain moist.

  3. The layer of muscles called the muscularis which squeezes the food down the oesophagus

  4. The adventitia keeps the oesophagus connected to the body through tissue, nerves, and smaller blood vessels.

  If you experience a sudden burning sensation in your chest, it can quite often be linked to problems such as acid reflux where a leaky muscle is more often the cause, allowing acid to leak into your oesophagus from the stomach.

- Stomach—your stomach is where most foods get properly digested and broken down. Hydrochloric acid, together with digestive enzymes, are released by the stomach the moment your brain acknowledges that you are about to eat. Your stomach pH can go as low as 1.5 when hydrochloric acid is released meaning it enters a very acidic state. The food mixed with stomach acid and enzymes turns into a half-liquid-like substance which is called *chyme* that then passes to the small intestines.

It's important for your stomach acid to reach the correct pH level to break down proteins in your food. This type of finer digestion is what allows the nutrients in food to get better absorbed into your bloodstream.

- Small intestine—as the chyme moves into the small intestine, its acidic levels are reduced by the emulsifying effects of bile secreted from the gallbladder and enzymes from your pancreas.

Part of your digestive and endocrine system includes the following glands.

- Liver
- Gallbladder
- Pancreas

Blood from the gut passes through the liver which then filters out toxins, stores any nutrients there, and helps to metabolise medication. The liver also secretes bile, which is stored in the gallbladder and released when needed.

Bile contains several substances and bilirubin is one; it is a waste product created by your red blood cells and is responsible for turning your stools the brownish colour they are most of the time. A light-coloured stool could indicate your food did not mix well with bile, which may be due to insufficient secretions.

- The bile and enzymes mix well with chyme/food as it is pushed through the small intestines, which like your oesophagus, has muscles that perform an action called *peristalsis*—an automatic contraction of the muscles in your GI tract to push food along.

- Also, as peristalsis takes place, the pancreatic enzymes will then work on proteins, carbs, and fats to break them down further to be absorbed into the small intestines.

As the food moves through your small intestines, it is exposed to tiny nodules called *villi*, that look like fingers lining the insides of the intestines. Villi makes absorption better and easier for the nutrients in the food you ate to enter your bloodstream. Villi are very thin and very sensitive and can be easily damaged.

Proper digestion is essential for the upper-digestive tract to ensure maximum absorption of nutrients. Also, that food must include a range of nutrients from all the food groups because eating the wrong foods can heavily impact the fine balance of digestion and absorption leading to ill health.

Apart from the wrong food, other factors that affect your digestive tract include illness and diseases, stress and anxiety, a lack of proper exercise, different types of medication, and ageing. Problems in the upper-digestive tract can influence the lower digestive tract as well, making it important to take care of stage one of your digestive system as a primary focus.

Signs Your Upper Digestive Tract is Not Okay

These are symptoms related to our gut, such as intermittent stomach pains, bloating, and gas we often experience, that we categorise as severe or mild. The latter is chosen often, with us dismissing or putting off investigating the reasons.

But that should not be the case because they are signals your upper-digestive tract is sending to let you know that all is not well. I have listed some of the common symptoms you may experience as a result of a problem with the normal function of your upper-digestive tract.

Feeling Full Soon After a Meal

This may be a symptom you experience on and off, feeling full soon after a meal even though you have eaten very little.

Feeling Bloated After a Meal

You feel full longer than you should after a meal. A feeling which continues long after you have eaten with bloating of the upper abdomen accompanied by an uncomfortable feeling of tightness in the stomach.

Pain and Unease in the Abdomen

You experience pain starting from your breastbone to your naval. It is an unsettling kind of pain that can keep changing from mild to severe.

Acid Reflux/Heartburn

A burning sensation in your upper abdomen is often caused by acid reflux which happens as a result of acid leaking back up from your stomach. It is often a burning sensation you feel starting from near the naval to a point below your breastbone.

Headaches too are often accompanied by this burning sensation which may or may not make you feel nauseous at the same time.

Nausea

Feeling nauseous as though you want to vomit. It is a prevailing feeling you may get both soon and long after a meal.

Gas

Gas is often caused by indigestion, disease, or bacteria in your digestive tract. Flatulence is common in this case which is the passing of gas from your anus.

Belching, which is the expulsion of air/gas from your mouth, may accompany flatulence or even occur on its own soon after you've eaten and may last long after.

What Can You Do to Ensure Optimal Health of Your Upper GI?

1. Support the secretion of your digestive enzymes called gastric secretion

Do this by ensuring you eat a balanced nutrient-dense meal, thus ensuring you provide your body with a good balance of essential macro and micronutrients vital for the proper secretion of digestive enzymes.

Your small intestines, stomach, and pancreas all produce digestive enzymes. The process takes place in three phases.

The cephalic phase—is the start of the phase when you put food in your mouth and your salivary glands start to secrete digestive enzymes.

The gastric phase—is the stage at which food reaches your stomach and starts to get broken down by stomach acids.

The Intestinal phase—at this stage your intestines secrete several enzymes including bicarbonate which diffuses the acidic component of the food.

Each one of these phases relies on vitamins and minerals to help it function and secrete enzymes at satisfactory levels that aid proper digestion.

How to Support the Secretion of Digestive Enzymes

- Amylase is a type of protein enzyme that is secreted by your salivary glands in your mouth and your pancreas. When secreted in your mouth, it helps to break down carbs. You can encourage the secretion of this protein by chewing your food thoroughly and giving it time to mix with the enzyme while breaking it down into small particles. Eating adequate numbers of protein will benefit the secretion of amylase.

- Hydrochloric acid is secreted from parietal cells in your stomach which need zinc to function. Therefore, zinc is an especially important micronutrient, because a deficiency of the mineral can lead to a reduction of stomach acid which in turn leads to poor digestion.

- Pancreatic juices which are a part of your digestive enzymes, help to break down starch, sugar, and fat in food. Secreted into the small intestine during the digestive process, pancreatic juices rely on vitamin D.

14

While our bodies produce only a minute percentage of the vitamin, we can obtain plenty from sunlight hitting our skins causing a synthesis process to produce vitamin D.

Your pancreas is also responsible for producing a range of hormones that influence the secretion of insulin which helps metabolise blood sugar. Glucagon signals the liver to release glucose stored there whenever your blood sugar levels go down. Amylin influences your appetite while gastrin aids with the secretion of stomach acids.

- Apple cider vinegar, lemon, papaya, and pineapple are considered supplements that influence the secretion of digestive enzymes. Make it a habit to drink a glass of water, mixed with lemon juice or a tablespoon of apple cider vinegar first thing when you wake to jump-start the secretion of your digestive enzymes. Likewise, eating food such as papaya and pineapple will help with the digestive process because these foods both contain naturally occurring enzymes that help with digestion.

Papaya and pineapple contain proteolytic enzymes that aid digestion and are produced in your pancreas and stomach. An enzyme called bromelain in pineapple and papain in papaya are types of proteolytic enzymes.

Additionally, you can ask your healthcare provider about taking digestive supplements. Proteolytic supplements are available as single-dose supplements meaning they contain a proteolytic from one source (eg, papaya) or it can be a mix of several types of digestive enzymes such as trypsin, pancreatin, papain, and bromelain.

15

- Eat slowly. Gulping down your food is not going to encourage the proper secretion of stomach acids. Eating too fast leads to bloating because you end up swallowing too much air. Slow and steady eating where your food is well-chewed, encourages the secretion of digestive enzymes throughout your upper GI.

2. Eat nutrient-dense food

Your body needs a combination of macro and micronutrients to survive at its fittest. That means including plenty of carbs, protein, fats, minerals, and vitamins in your diet.

Age too, is another factor affecting digestion because as we age, our body's ability to produce essential vitamins and minerals depletes, making it important to supplement ourselves through our diet. With age, the performance of the pancreas starts to reduce causing several shortcomings in the secretion of enzymes, bile, and other functions related to digestion.

You will be surprised to learn that your GI performance starts to decline as early as age 20, making it imperative that parents ensure their children maintain their gut health.

The Lower-Digestive System—Stage Two

This section consists of the large intestine which is made up of the colon, rectum, and the anus, which is basically one long tube, thicker than the small intestine. It begins where the small intestine ends, signalling the end of the digestion process.

The Colon: Quite often the term colon will be used to mean your large intestine where the liquid from semi-solid bits of food passed down from the small intestines is absorbed turning them into solid stools to be expelled from your anus.

The point at which digested food enters the colon from the small intestines is called the *cecum* which is about six inches in length. The cecum is like a sealed sack located inside the colon. It is connected to the small intestine and when filled with the digested food, will induce muscle contractions in the colon to pass the food along.

If you recall pictures of your long intestine, you'd remember that it coils around the small intestines, which are located in the middle. Thus, food travels to the upper part of the long intestine/colon where most or all of the liquid and electrolytes are absorbed. And as the food is then pushed downward heading toward the anus it is already in a solid form.

Solids move through the colon easily because of the mucus that's secreted. Again, digestion takes place of the remaining food particles but this time through the influence of your gut bacteria and not enzymes. The good bacteria in your microbiota break down food to absorb essential vitamins and minerals that are fat-soluble; gut bacteria break down food particles through fermentation. Vitamins produced through the influence of your gut bacteria include B-vitamins, vitamin K and biotin. As you would have guessed this fermentation process of digestion takes much longer than digestion influenced by enzymes in your upper digestive tract.

The Rectum: Once all the nutrients are absorbed, just about all of the liquid that remains of the food you ate will enter the rectum. This substance now looks like regular poop and will contain waste material your body wishes to get rid of. This is mainly the husks of what you ate or rather the parts that cannot be digested, waste from your intestinal mucus that gets accumulated along the way, dead cells, and some water as well as mucus. What you are ready to poop now is a little less than a quarter of the food that was passed from the small intestines to the colon. And as muscles contract to allow food to enter the rectum you start to feel as though you need to defecate.

The Anus: This section is kind of like the airlocks you see on spaceships (in the movies of course). Each end of the anus is locked by what is called an *anal sphincter* which is really a muscle that contracts to open and close the entrance and exits of your anus which is the end section of the lower gut.

The two sphincters located on either side of the anus are a good thing because otherwise, you would have poop sliding right out of your rectum and through to your anus, Instead, you have these locks. You are in control of the opening of the external anal sphincter which lets out your poop.

The muscles on the internal sphincter relax and open when nerve signals are sent from your rectum to say that the waste has arrived thus letting in the stools to the anus. At the same time, your body alerts you about the need to use the toilet. Once the poop enters the anus it stays locked inside until you relax the external anal sphincter to let out your body's waste material.

Maintaining the Health of Your Lower-Digestive System—Home to Your Microbiota

There are many theories about the number of bacteria in your microbiome. And for a long time, it was believed the microbiome consisted of tenfold the number of cells in your body. However, research shows the number is most likely at a 1:1 ratio of bacteria to cells in your body (Sender et al., 2016). But none of these findings deters from the importance of your microbiome which is the collection of good and bad bacteria in your gut. The various tasks and influences the good bacteria in your gut microbiome are responsible for are invaluable toward your overall health. Thus, compounding the importance of taking care of your lower digestive system.

Why Is Gut Bacteria So Important?

Your gut microbiome consists of bacteria, viruses, and fungi that thrive inside your body internally and externally on your skin.

The gut microbiota which lives in your lower-GI tract is made up of bacteria and archaea which are single-celled organisms that have origins dating back to early life. Therefore, some types of bacteria we harbour in our microbiome have evolved over time with us.

While a baby is born with a healthy microbiota, there are external factors too that influence the quality of a person's good gut bacteria. And it is important to maintain a healthy balance of your gut microbiota as it influences your immune system, metabolism, digestive tract, and your nervous system.

But together with the good services, your gut bacteria perform there are those that cause illness and disease.

- Obesity, cancer, diabetes, heart ailments, and colitis are some of the negative effects bad gut bacteria can have on your health

The beneficial effects of your gut microbiota are many.

- Helping ferment undigested intestinal mucus and food particles, especially dietary fibres that the upper digestive tract cannot break down, is one of the important functions of your gut bacteria.

- Strengthening your immune system, optimising nutrition, and fighting disease are some of the benefits we rely on maintaining through our gut bacteria.

Chapter 2 is all about your gut microbiome, where you can learn more about the importance of these microorganisms for

19

your overall health. But for now, it's important to establish that your microbiota is the most important element of your lower digestive tract.

Identifying Problems With Your Lower-Digestive System

Keeping your gut microbiome healthy is essential for your overall health and wellbeing. Therefore, problems in your lower-digestive system should not be taken lightly. Problems with the lower-digestive system can be related to several reasons. The food you ate, a family history of gut disease, stress, and bacteria are some.

Symptoms and causes to watch out for include the following.

- Irritable bowel syndrome (IBS) frequently affects the large intestines. Gas and indigestion, which can cause swelling around your belly button, may be due to IBS and also an imbalance of the gut microbiome.

- Abdominal inflammation of the colon and the rectum could be an indication of ulcerative colitis that can occur when very small ulcers appear on the lining of the colon; pus and blood will sometimes leak from them.

- Crohn's disease or inflammatory bowel disease (IBD) can cause symptoms of diarrhoea, abdominal pain, weight loss, and fatigue.

- Fatigue can also be due to a problem in the gut microbiome due to bacteria or a virus or dangerous microorganisms in the gut.

- Mood swings can occur due to reasons that disrupt your gut-brain axis; thus, causing alterations in your mood. Such disruptions can lead to an inflamed nervous system which is often due to depression or anxiety issues.

- Bloating around the belly button could be due to gas and indigestion or even a problem with your gut microbiome.

- SIBO is bacterial growth in your small intestines which is an overgrowth of bacteria in the small intestines; these bacterial types are not common to the small intestines. Symptoms include loss of appetite, nausea, bloating, diarrhoea. Sudden weight loss and lasting diarrhoea and stomach pain symptoms must be medically checked for SIBO.

Simple Habits to Keep Your Lower-Digestive System Healthy

There are some methods you can use to help your lower-digestive system stay fit. Keep in mind that a majority of problems in your digestive tract can be attributed to your lifestyle. Because while our diets have evolved to include a range of processed foods that are far from their natural state our digestive systems have not. Our biological systems too are struggling to cope with modern habits; too much time on tech devices, late nights, and loads of stress leading to depression. These are all factors that lead to problems in your gut.

Maintain the Health of Your Gut Bacteria

Starve the bad bacteria in your gut. You can do this by ensuring you eat a nutritionally-dense diet. Leave out the added-sugar treats and the processed foods. Bad bacteria in your gut microbiome thrive on sugar and the last thing you need to do is encourage the growth of bad bacteria.

Fermented food and food containing prebiotics are highly beneficial to the good bacteria in your gut, thus, maintaining a healthy balance; both contain good bacteria and will supplement your gut flora to ensure the ratio of good bacteria remains high.

Popular options for fermented food include the following which can be store-bought or made at home. Starter culture, which is the bacteria you add to ferment the food can be bought according to the needs that each strain of the bacteria caters to.

- Kimchi is a side dish you can order from your favourite Korean restaurant. You can also make it at home as it contains vegetables, fish sauce, salt and spices that are left to ferment in jars. You can make it and store it as needed.

  Kimchi contains three beneficial bacteria. Weissella for anti-inflammatory and antibiotic properties, lactobacillus that's found in yoghurt, and leuconostoc, a popular starter culture.

- kombucha, is a probiotic fizzy drink made by fermenting tea, and sugar with a gut-healthy bacterial culture and yeast. The bacteria ferments the drink by eating the sugar to make a delicious and healthy drink. Extended fermentation times make the drink more fizzy and tasty.

- Sauerkraut can be bought ready-made or can be homemade. Made by fermenting vegetables over time, sauerkraut too can be stored.

- Coconut yoghurt is an ideal substitute for dairy and can also be home made with a starter culture.

- Kefir, made with kefir grains and cow milk, is a popular fermented drink originating from Russia. A good antibacterial too, kefir grains contain good bacteria that ferment the milk. The longer it's kept to ferment the richer the taste.

*Do not eat fermented food if you are dealing with SIBO.

Prebiotics is a type of dietary fibre that is food for the good bacteria in your gut. Consider prebiotics as fertiliser for your good bacteria which helps it thrive. Complex fibres found in fruits and vegetables

- Banana
- Chicory
- Asparagus
- Onions
- Leeks
- Apples
- Artichoke
- Barley
- Cocoa

Bone broth too is highly beneficial to your gut bacteria as it contains several vitamins and minerals including glutamine, glycine, gelatin, and collagen some of the trace minerals and amino acids needed for strengthening your immune system and creating a strong barrier thus preventing toxins from leaking into your bloodstream.

Supplement on probiotics. These are essentially good bacteria you are adding to your microbiome. Probiotics also thrive in food such as yoghurt and help to maintain a good balance of your gut microbiome.

Drink plenty of liquids. Fluids are a great asset to your overall health. Staying well hydrated will ensure your digestive tract works at its optimal best.

Making a conscious effort to change your lifestyle habits will have a huge impact on the health of your digestive system. Picking and choosing the right type of food will not only keep your gut healthy, but in time, will reset some chronic illnesses you may be dealing with. It's important to think about your overall health as beginning from your gut and so, we will use the next chapter to learn more about the bacteria that thrive in your gut.

Chapter 2:

A Closer Look at Your Gut Microbiome

We are now going to explore in detail the importance of your gut microbiome, thus reconfirming the importance of this huge system of microorganisms which is really an entire organ on its own containing all the viruses, bacteria, and fungi in your biological system.

While some of the bacteria that make up your gut microbiome are harmful, the rest perform invaluable functions from curing and preventing a number of diseases to aiding and strengthening your immune system, digestion, weight management, appetite, mood regulation, and heart health. Getting to know your gut microbiome can be complicated; not only is it made up of close to 100 trillion bacteria, but its many functions are vast and some are still a mystery to researchers.

What Is Your Gut Microbiome?

A large portion of bacteria, the bacteria that exist on your skin and internally, live in your digestive tract and make up your gut microbiome; a majority live in your large intestines as their main function is to aid your digestive process by breaking down and absorbing the nutrients from the food you eat. There are over 1,000 variants of bacteria that make up your gut or intestinal microbiome.

In conjunction, the good bugs in your gut bacteria will help with the following:

- Synthesise your food while further working on the particles that remain after the digestive process of the upper GI. The bacteria work by breaking them down to the smallest possible particles for optimal absorption.
- Prevent the regurgitation of food or acid reflux.
- Helps you to have regular bowel movements.
- Stop the discomfort of bloating.
- Help reduce the occurrence of food allergies.

The digestive process is not all your gut microbiome is responsible for; the gut microbiome also functions as an extension to your endocrine system which is responsible for the regularisation of your hormone secretion.

The endocrine system is made up of glands that secrete chemicals that act as hormone neurotransmitters; your gut microbiome, likewise, releases several chemicals to your bloodstream which influence a range of functions ranging from helping control your mood to your appetite. The gut-brain connection is what aids this function with your gut bacteria having the power to influence the function of your brain.

What Makes Your Gut Bacteria Unique?

The gut microbiome of each person is different; so different that not even identical twins share 100% of the same microbiome pattern. In contrast, there is a 99.9% similarity between the DNA of two people, which makes your gut microbiome even more special and unique.

The gut bacteria combination between individuals is so unique that the similarity of the gut microbiome is only 34% between identical twins and 30% between unrelated individuals (Berry et al., 2020). This huge difference between your gut microbiome signature is due to genetics, with each person possessing different strains of microorganisms.

On this same line, each one of us belongs to a specific *enterotype*, which is how living organisms are grouped based on the bacterial community they possess in their gut microbiome.

Scientists have found three enterotypes, or groups, that people can be classified into based on the specific bacterial cluster types found in their microbiome; the types of bacteria present are often determined by a person's diet.

The three enterotypes are as follows.

1. Bacteroides—the specific type of bacterial microorganisms present in this classification were found more among people who ate a diet rich in animal fats and protein.

2. Prevotella—the most common types of bacterial microorganisms found in this group were shared among people whose diets were more carb-based, akin to plant food.

3. Ruminococcus—the type of bacterial organisms found in this group are similar to those present in the bacteroid classification with people in this group exhibiting similar dietary patterns.

What's interesting are the connections researchers have made among the bacterial clusters and diets the people belonging to each group followed.

In both the bacteroid and ruminococcus enterotypes, bacterial organisms that encourage lipid metabolization were greater, while the frequency of the same bacterial organisms found among the prevotella group was greater among people following a vegetarian diet. This confirms that microorganisms have preferences and react differently to varied types of food.

Another important finding was the reduction of what is known as commensal bacteria in patients diagnosed with IBD (F. Moraes et al., 2019). Commensal bacteria work to strengthen the immune system as a kind of forcefield by preventing the colonisation and invasion of foreign organisms that can cause disease, further proving the importance of your gut bacteria in preventing disease.

How Is Your Gut Microbiome Determined?

Your gut microbiome started to form when you were in the womb. And as you grew, the bacterial lifeforms there grew and evolved. A large part of your gut microbiome is predetermined and cannot be changed. Factors that influence your gut microbiome include the following:

- Genetics plays a part in pre-determining your gut microbiome.
- Parental health at the time of conception.
- Delivery type, whether vaginal or caesarean, makes a difference because babies born through their mother's birth canal become exposed to more bacteria there and have a more diverse gut microbiome than those born through a c-section.

- Factors such as being breastfed or bottle-fed too have the same effects as birth type with breastfed babies becoming more exposed to different strains of bacteria as opposed to bottle-fed babies who are fed through sterilised bottle teats.
- The environment you grew up in can help shape your gut microbiome. For example, an over-sterile environment that prevents you from being exposed to different strains of bacteria will prevent you from becoming exposed to various viruses and bacteria, thus preventing your gut microbiome too from experiencing and building resilience against different types of bacteria.

These markers that influence your gut microbiome may not be within your control, but others such as lifestyle and diet are and play an equally important role in influencing the health and performance of your gut microbiome.

Maintaining the Health of Your Gut Microbiome

The two main factors that determine your gut health are your intestinal microbiome and your gut barrier. If either one is compromised, you face an imbalance and malfunction of important tasks your gut bacteria perform.

The gut barrier refers to the mucosa or mucous membrane located inside your intestines; it's there to prevent the leakage of food particles and bacterial and viral compounds that can get into your bloodstream and cause damage.

The health of your gut microbiome is measured by the diversity of the microorganisms living there, how strong that microbial community is, and its resilience toward change that could alter its environment. Dysbiosis is a condition that occurs when that delicate balance is disrupted.

Dysbiosis

It is considered healthy to have a diverse variety of bacteria inhabiting your gut microbiome; while the bad bugs can cause harm, the good bugs in your gut microbiome are needed to help you stay healthy. Through exterior influences, of which food is one of the key influencers, the fine balance between the good and bad bacteria can go off, leading to unhealthy results. Such harmful effects on the gut microbiome that put the system off balance leads to what is called *dysbiosis*.

Factors Leading to Dysbiosis

There are several reasons leading to dysbiosis:

- Eating the wrong type of food or sudden changes in your diet to include more protein, processed foods, artificial sweeteners, and added sugars. Eating too much protein is linked to diseases such as colorectal cancer which can occur when too much protein sits and ferments in the large intestines, which in turn, induces the release of harmful metabolites produced from certain strains of bacteria.

- Antibiotics can harm and put your gut flora out of balance. Also, eating meat products from livestock that were raised on antibiotics can have similar effects. Antibiotics are taken to get rid of bad gut bacteria but some can affect good bacteria too, causing a change to the balance of your gut microbiome that is not favourable to your health.

- Medication. In addition to antibiotics causing harm to your good gut bacteria, there are some medicine types that can cause harm. Medications taken as anti-acid reflux solutions, certain painkillers you can buy over the counter, drugs taken to combat diabetes, and medicine prescribed for anxiety and mood disorders.

- Consuming more than one alcoholic drink a day may lead to alcohol dependency and eventually addiction. Alcohol disrupts the balance of your gut microbiome with research proving the point that the gut microbiome of alcoholics is different from the average person (Mutlu et al., 2012). The growth of harmful bacteria is encouraged by the overconsumption of alcohol, with some that cause liver damage starting to thrive, fatty liver too occurs due to alcohol induced fat deposits in the liver.

- Eating fruits or vegetables that have traces of chemicals (from fertiliser). Pesticides can cause serious harm to your gut bacteria; that is apart from the fertility, neurological and respiratory problems it causes. Glyphosate, which is a chemical compound used to kill weeds, can be especially harmful to your gut microbiome. Some studies suggest the compound may be carcinogenic to people, which means it can cause cancers. Studies have also revealed that glyphosate alters the gut microbiome environment which too can lead to dysbiosis (Nielsen et al., 2018).

- Improper dental care encourages the growth of bad bacteria in your mouth. This happens when you neglect your oral hygiene routines, thus allowing bad bacteria to thrive. Thoroughly washing all produce in running water before cooking or consuming them raw, is the best practice. In the case of hard vegetables or fruits, get used to scrubbing them with a vegetable brush to ensure you get rid of all the surface contaminants.

- Unprotected sexual intercourse exposes you to bad bacteria and viruses. Any type of sexual activity results in the transfer of viruses, bacteria, and fungi between individuals. Thus, causing an invasion and an imbalance in the gut flora.

- The weakening of your immune system is caused by stress and anxiety. This can happen when your good gut bacteria is affected, inhibiting the production of a substance known as immunoglobulin A (IgA), a type of antibody protein that is found mainly in the gut mucus membrane. Some percentages are also present in the respiratory tract, saliva, tears, and breastmilk. IgA helps fight infections that can occur due to toxins that enter your body but are affected by autoimmune diseases/conditions such as IBS and leaky gut. Studies have confirmed that prolonged negative thoughts and stress can affect the production of IgA (Campos-Rodríguez, 2013).

- Leading an Inactive Lifestyle

As surprising as this may sound to you, becoming accustomed to a sedentary lifestyle can have detrimental effects on your gut microbiome. If you spend a major portion of your day sitting or lying down you can classify yourself as leading a sedentary lifestyle.

Did you know that it is against your good health to sit for more than three hours a day? Sitting for up to four hours a day is ranked as low risk and sitting for eight hours or more is ranked as leading a high-risk lifestyle.

Being active has positive effects on your gut flora; where an active lifestyle encourages the growth of bacteria that produces a short chain fatty acid called butyrate. The substance is needed to maintain your gut health and to energise the cells in your gut. Butyrate is the least produced fatty acid in your system, therefore, getting out of your chair and going for a brisk walk, or jog is going to encourage the production of this much-needed nutrient.

How to Identify Dysbiosis

Symptoms of dysbiosis can change depending on the type of bad bacteria that are thriving in your gut. Some of the general symptoms will include the following:

- Diarrhoea
- Constipation
- Bloating
- Bad breath (halitosis)
- Feeling nauseous
- Pain in the chest
- Feeling bloated
- Itching in the vagina or rectum
- Sudden rashes or red patches
- Feeling tired that's out of the ordinary
- Anxiety and depression

If you are dealing with any of these symptoms, it's important to visit your healthcare provider to have them checked out. There are several testing methods used to diagnose dysbiosis such as the hydrogen breath test which tests your breath for the presence of types of gases that are produced by bacteria, a urine acidity test, and testing of the stools.

What are the Risk Factors of Acquiring Dysbiosis

Dysbiosis has been linked to several syndromes and diseases that can be caused by a disruption of your gut microbiome's normal function. Some of them may develop and affect areas/organs outside of your GI tract or may be conditions that occur as a result of a hormonal imbalance caused by a disruption of your gut microbiome. Some will directly affect your intestines.

- Obesity

- Diabetes

- Disease in the liver

- Development of cancer in the colon or rectum

- Candida, a yeast infection

- Eczema and other skin conditions

- The development of dementia or Parkinson's

- Leaky gut syndrome

- Irritable bowel syndrome (IBS)

The last two directly affect the quality and function of your GI tract.

Dysbiosis and Leaky Gut Syndrome

Types of calorie-dense, highly-processed foods that also contain emulsifiers/additives (which are added to help combine certain food types like oil and water that simply do not mix), can cause harm to the delicate balance of your gut flora leading to a break in the mucus barrier of your intestinal wall allowing toxins to leak into your bloodstream and into your gut. While there are several, one of the main causes for the development of a leaky gut is dysbiosis.

With dysbiosis, this becomes easier because your good bacteria count is lowered and bad bacteria starts to thrive, the release of what's called enterotoxins takes place.

This is a type of protein compound released by certain types of harmful bacteria that is also responsible for causing syndromes such as food poisoning. Keep in mind that bad bacteria may even become stronger when encouraged to feed off the types of unhealthy foods mentioned above; processed meats and dairy have a higher probability of containing bacteria that produce enterotoxins.

Owing to these causes, most people end up with a gut that leaks food particles and bacteria into their bloodstream, thus ending up being diagnosed with a leaky gut which is a syndrome often associated with autoimmune diseases such as chronic inflammation.

Leaky Gut and Chronic Inflammation

Chronic inflammation occurs when your own immune system starts to attack your cells because with a leaky gut your intestines lose their mucus shield and becomes permeable allowing toxins into your bloodstream and back into your gut, and so, your immune system starts to overwork to fight the invaders. Plus you lose a large chunk of nutrients that seep through before your intestines can absorb them making you weaker.

Your immune system automatically secretes inflammatory cytokines, a protein substance that binds with cells to form a barrier or to eliminate infected cells which can become damaged by bacterial infections or trauma, either caused by foreign particles or from injuries. The result is acute inflammation at the damaged site which subsides once the area is cleansed or healed.

This is a natural defence mechanism your body adapts to keep you safe from foreign invasions, and injuries. But when leaky gut becomes a syndrome your immune system goes into overdrive where a constant release of cytokines and inflammatory cells eventually leads to a condition called chronic inflammation, meaning the automatic inflammatory response from your immune system remains constant which in turn causes your own immune system to start attacking your healthy cells as a result.

Symptoms of Leaky Gut

There is no hard and fast rule to say the symptoms I am listing here are always associated with a leaky gut. But this is generally how the condition is diagnosed.

- Too much bloating and gas are caused by an overgrowth of bad bacteria.

- Since mucosa gets leaked out from your gut, digestion becomes painful.

- Experiencing a burning sensation in your gut as though you are suffering from ulceration.

- Diarrhoea

- A zap in your energy levels since food is leaked out before all the nutrients can be absorbed.

Can I Be Dealing With Leaky Gut Syndrome?

A leaky gut causes both your gut to leak and also become permeable which means substances can leak back into your gut. If you suspect you may be dealing with the syndrome, here are common symptoms that should alert you to seek medical help.

- Development of food sensitivities

- Pain in your abdomen

- Indigestion

- Bloating

In addition to these symptoms, the erosion of your intestinal walls will have other effects where not only is your immune system challenged and weakened but your digestion process will start to suffer. At the same time, the levels of pain sensitivity in your intestines are going to increase leaving you with an overall uneasy feeling that everything is not A-okay.

Dysbiosis can be cured and is often quite mild at the start. That is why it's important to have any symptoms, especially stomach pains, sudden rashes, or skin conditions that crop up, checked by a healthcare provider. While the condition can be treated with medication, simple lifestyle changes that include avoiding the factors that lead to the development of dysbiosis can sometimes cure, as well as, prevent the occurrence of the condition.

Conditions Associated With Leaky Gut

The medical conditions I have listed below are associated with leaky gut syndrome, however, they are not conclusive evidence you have a leaky gut and could be experienced as an independent disease. This is why proper medical diagnosis is important in case you identify any symptoms of leaky gut.

- Celiac disease also called coeliac disease
- Chronic liver disease
- IBS
- Diabetes
- Rheumatoid arthritis
- Psoriasis
- Chronic fatigue
- Crohn's disease
- Food sensitivities and allergies
- Nutritional deficiencies
- Polycystic ovarian syndrome (POS)
- Premenstrual syndrome

Manage Leaky Gut Syndrome With Simple Lifestyle Changes

Managing or avoiding conditions like leaky gut, can sometimes be accomplished with simple lifestyle changes. And while I have already listed the reasons that lead to dysbiosis which is the main cause of leaky gut, I will stress once more the importance of adopting the following as a way to deal with the leaky gut condition.

- Stop smoking, if you find this a chore, seek medical help. There are several remedies you can use to gradually curtail and eventually stop your habit of smoking which in truth is a cause of many degenerative diseases like cancers.

- Control your alcohol intake. A drink to relax, celebrate or spend time with friends is fine (unless of course you have been medically advised to stay off alcohol). If not, consciously curtailing your alcohol consumption will help you to continue enjoying an occasional drink and safeguard your wellbeing.

- Enjoy an active lifestyle. Exercise or indulge in some form of physical exertion that you enjoy. Avoid a sedentary lifestyle.

- Reduce your stress. Find methods to deal with your anxiety, share your burdens, and do not overburden your mind. Make it a habit to decompress and destress at the end of the day. Enjoy time on your own, make time to take care of your needs, and savour life in slow motion avoiding the rush.

- Get enough sleep. Try to add at least seven to eight hours of quality sleep to your nightly schedule. Avoid late hours watching television and make bedtime a set timetable so you teach your body to follow a proper sleep-wake cycle.

- Consider your diet. Avoid added sugars and artificial sweeteners. Include plenty of fibre and probiotics.

The Food You Eat Has a Major Impact on Your Gut Microbiome

Your diet is most likely varied and consists of different types of food; whether you are a vegan, vegetarian, or follow a paleo diet, amongst others, makes no difference, you will most likely be eating food from varied sources.

There are certain types of food that have a particular effect on your gut microbiome, offering both positive and negative benefits. Some feed the good bacteria in your gut helping the micro-organisms thrive and carry out their many important tasks.

Other food types are harmful and will put your gut bacteria off balance and encourage bad bacteria to outnumber the good. They can impact your gut bacteria so strongly that in time, your microbial signature or your enterotype will evolve to become one that leads to conditions such as IBS, obesity, and other conditions governed mostly by the health of your gut.

Foods that cause an impact on your gut microbiome include dietary fibres, dietary fats, animal products, and artificial sweeteners. It is important to include a diverse variety of food in your diet to encourage the many types of micro-organisms living in your gut because let's not forget that the more diverse your gut bacteria is, the more beneficial the system is to your overall health.

How to Improve Your Gut Bacteria Through Food

1. Change your dietary patterns to include diverse food types

It's important to eat food from various sources and different food groups. There must be a healthy balance of plant food too, that you can obtain from diverse groups. Unfortunately, the typical western diet which has evolved over time to include a variety of artificial ingredients and highly processed food types, limits the number of natural plant and animal food we consume, thus restricting the diversity of nutrients you supply to your gut microbiome. Further compounding this fact, is research that links the richness of the gut microbiome to a diverse diet (Heiman & Greenway, 2016).

Here are some tips to diversify your diet because the quality of your gut microbiome depends on the quality of the food you eat.

- Choose fruits and vegetables in a variety of colours. This is one way of ensuring you feed your intestinal bacteria with a range of nutrients. Phytonutrients, also known as polyphenols, are a natural compound present in plant food and are responsible for lending fruits and vegetables their myriad colours.

  Phytonutrients are a type of prebiotic, and therefore act as a fertiliser for your gut bacteria. The compound feeds a type of gut bacteria called Bifidobacteria. This strain of bacteria is highly vital to your wellbeing as they help fight infections, aid with the digestion of dietary fibres, and produce essential vitamin K, B vitamins, and fatty acids. Aim to eat at least five different-coloured fruits and vegetables a day as each colour offers a specific range of benefits.

2. Try eating seasonal vegetables and fruits

Another way to add variety to your diet and also enjoy creating a diverse range of dishes is to choose to eat seasonal fruits and vegetables. We often tend to stick to the same old food groups because those types of plant food are available throughout the year and can be easily incorporated into our ritual recipes.

Benefits of seasonal vegetables:

- There is no shipping contamination as you are eating produce that's homegrown.
- Seasonal produce is fresher.
- Supportive and environment friendly because local farmers are supported and you eat what the land yields minus transport costs and pollution.
- Supports your body's nutritional needs; for example, winter vegetables make excellent comfort meals like soups.

As the most important system in your body, your gut certainly deserves a whole lot of tender love and care. To do this, you need to be in tune with your GI tract and not take your digestive process as an automatic function.

Think of your gut as the fuel distribution unit of a luxury car. The car is your body and it will only perform at its optimum best, offering you a smooth ride, when fed with A-grade fuel, and managed through regular services and proper maintenance.

Similarly, you must be in tune with your body by being able to identify when your gut is healthy and when it is having problems. There are several signals your body sends out that all is not well with your GI tract. And because your gut impacts all areas of your bodily functions, your organs, and cells and is

42

therefore responsible for your overall health, it's crucial you pay attention to your gut health.

How to Know Your Gut is Healthy

You already know that there are several factors that determine your gut health ranging from eating the wrong type of food to stress and too much alcohol to the use of antibiotics that can affect the delicate balance of your intestinal microbiome which in turn disrupts the function of your digestive tract.

If there are no outwardly signs, how do you know your GI tract is healthy or having problems?

You may not be aware of them but there are several signals and signs your body sends to let you know that all is not well with your digestive system. Likewise, there are simple habits you can adopt to keep a check on your most important biological system. I am talking about everyday habits like checking your poop (just a simple glance into the toilet will do), and eating food that's gut healthy. Let's start with the closest representation of how well your digestive tract is doing—your poop!

1. Learn to Read Your Poop

Before you go "eww", let me remind you that your poop is your outward representative of what's actually happening inside of your digestive system. In other words, what you reap is what you sow in terms of the type of poop that your body expels, and learning to read your poop is one of the best methods to stay updated about your overall health.

Not all poop is the same, if you take the time to give your poop a second glance before you flush it away, you will realise that there are changes in texture, colour, and pooping frequency, depending on what you ate, and how healthy or sick you are as well as the levels of stress you are dealing with.

What Is Poop Made of?

It is of course the waste products expelled from your body once your GI tract has absorbed all the nutrients. But what exactly is the composition of poop? It may not be a pretty sight but it's important to know what your poop contains.

Here is a list of what is in your poop (Britannica, 2019).

- Almost 75% of your stools are made up of water.
- Solids make up the balance 25%
    - Food particles that never get digested, which consist mostly of fibres as they are the hardest for your digestive system to break down but are needed for the formation of healthy easy-to-pass stools, as well as indigestible substances like cellulose.
    - Waste that your body is expelling; fats such as cholesterol as well as red blood cells that have been used which lend the brownish colour to your poop as they get mixed with bile before being expelled by the liver as a substance called *bilirubin*.
    - Dead bacteria from your microbiome make up about 30% of the solids in your stools.
    - Inorganic compounds like iron and calcium.

What Does Healthy Poop Look Like?

The only way to decipher your poop quality is to have a look at it. The consistency of your pooping schedule is a good indicator of your gut health but the shape, colour, and smell (yes, I said it) are all indicators of how healthy you are. Once you look beyond the 'gross' factor, you are going to realise how easy it is to keep check of your overall health by simply keeping a check on your poop, and in time checking your poop is going to become an automatic reflex for you.

Reading Into the Shape and Size of Your Poop

Have you heard of the Bristol Stool Scale? It is a medical tool/chart that healthcare providers use to gauge the quality of your stools. Below is an example of what the Bristol Scale looks like.

1	○○○○○	**Type 1** Separate hard lumps like nuts (difficult to pass)
2	⬭⬭⬭⬭	**Type 2** Sausage shaped but lumpy
3	⬭⬭⬭⬭	**Type 3** Like a sausage but with cracks on the surface
4	⌒	**Type 4** Like a sausage or snake smooth and soft
5	○ ○ ○	**Type 5** Soft blobs with clear-cut edges (passed easily)
6	⌇⌇⌇	**Type 6** Fluffy pieces with ragged edges, a mushy stool
7	～	**Type 7** Watery, no solid pieces (entirely liquid)

Type 1–2 which indicates hard pellets or several hard pieces lumped together to form a solid stool that's hard to pass and sometimes causes pain, which is most likely due to constipation that can occur due to dehydration and insufficient fibre in your diet.

Type 3–4 indicates normal healthy stools. They are medium-soft to firm and will have a smooth texture, as well as a sausage shape that may be deposited as one large single piece or broken into smaller pieces that will sink and sit at the bottom of the toilet bowl. Floaty stools indicate there is a higher percentage of fat that's undigested in them.

Type 5–7 are soft, mushy pieces or totally runny stools created by diarrhoea which can be due to several reasons such as bacteria, food sensitivities, digestive problems, and even side effects of certain medications.

How Colour Can Indicate the Health of Your Poop

Healthy poop will have brown tones, ranging from an earthy colour to sometimes light and dark shades of brown, let's not forget that bilirubin lends the brownish shades to your poop.

Sometimes, our poop changes colour and could indicate a mild to severe infection or disease. Let's look at what the different colours of your poop indicate.

Green—occasional green poop can occur if you've eaten a large amount of green plant food because the chlorophyll present in green plants can cause a change in the colour of your poop. The same can happen if you eat food made with green colouring.

Otherwise, poop can turn green if it contains higher numbers of bile than normal. This is normal if it is occasional but if bile causes green poop regularly it could indicate that your digestive process is working too fast and not allowing time for bile to be synthesised. Since you cannot tell, either way, it is important to visit your healthcare provider and have your concerns checked.

Another reason for poop turning green is an infection that can be caused by bacteria. Green stools are especially common when your gut is infected with the salmonella bacterium and Giardia which is a parasite found in water.

Red-hued poop—again eating food with red colouring or even vegetables like beetroot can cause red stools. But if you do notice reddish stools frequently even when you have not eaten red-coloured food, it could indicate some form of bleeding in your GI tract. If you have any concerns or something doesn't seem normal, then speak to your healthcare provider.

Black or very dark brownish stools—can be caused by an iron supplement you are taking or may be due to bleeding in your upper intestines. If you have any concerns or something doesn't seem normal, then speak to your healthcare provider.

Bright red stools—happen if there is bleeding in your lower-digestive system. The cause could be due to haemorrhoids. However, an occasional bright-red poop could be caused by red-coloured foods such as dyes, beets, or even tomatoes so you should not panic at the first sight of a red stool. If you have any concerns or something doesn't seem normal, then speak to your healthcare provider.

Clay-coloured or white stools—are a good indication of not enough bile in the system. Or it could be due to ingesting large quantities of antidiarrheal medications such as bismuth subsalicylate.

How Often Must You Poop?

You may be one, or you may know someone who has a very reliable pooping schedule and has a bowel movement at about the same time daily. On the flip side, there are others who have no bowel movements at all on some days. Which do you think is acceptable as healthy?

Surprisingly, either habit is acceptable. Let me remind you about how unique the gut microbiome is from person to person, likewise, we all share the same physical needs that take place on entirely different schedules.

While you may be able to hold in your urge to pee until you get home when you are out and about, your friend may need to visit public bathrooms more frequently, or vice versa. Therefore, you cannot gauge your poop schedule on someone else's habits.

Research has revealed that pooping schedules are indeed diverse among people, with some needing to poop two to three times a day, and others needing to pass stools only two to three times a week. These two alternate frequencies of bowel movements were reported among 96% of the subjects interviewed (Mitsuhashi et al., 2018). Which makes it safe to conclude that if it is your regular habit, there is no cause for concern.

Anything out of your ordinary pooping pattern must be considered a cause for concern. For example, a person who has a regular poop at least once a day should consider being constipated for several days as a cause for concern because constipation can be attributed to several causes.

Not having a bowel movement for more than three days a week is also a cause for concern; it could be due to several reasons such as stress, overdoing it with laxatives, or even more serious reasons such as anal fissures or haemorrhoids.

Factors that affect your bowel movements include the following:

- Diet
- The natural activity of your gut
- The capacity of your rectum
- Your lifestyle habits
- The health of your gut microbiome

The three bowel movements per day or per week being the accepted norm among a majority of people means health caregivers will show more concern about how much strain or pain you endure when passing stools over frequency.

Pooping With No Pain

Expelling your poop must be no hassle, it should be an easy smooth expulsion with no pain. Those are signs of a healthy gut. Having to push and strain or experience pain when pooping could mean several things such as constipation or even IBS. Either way, such symptoms are an alert that all is not well with your gut and you need to visit your healthcare provider for further investigations.

2. Bloating and Gas—When Is it Okay to Fart?

Gas is produced by the bacteria that make up your gut microbiome. It is a by-product created by the micro-organisms feeding on the food you supply them. Imagine trillions of bugs feeding and then releasing gases inside your digestive tract! Well, it must all escape or you will end up feeling uncomfortable and bloated.

Farting, as well as belching, as politely incorrect as many of us believe the act to be, is a necessary reflex that we must give in to (maybe discreetly and in private when possible).

It is natural for a person to fart up to 20 times a day, that is in fact a sign of a healthy gut. Gas or air builds up mostly when you are eating, released by your gut bacteria, and also when you swallow air, which happens naturally as you eat.

Excessive swallowing of air can occur due to lifestyle habits like smoking and drinking through a straw. While eating hard-to-digest food and dealing with stress, constipation and certain types of illness can cause excessive gas to form internally.

What if You Hold in a Fart?

There may be several times you have held in a fart because the timing was just not right to let out a potentially noisy or smelly expulsion of air from your anus.

You may have even swallowed a burp on occasion. Have you ever wondered if doing so could cause you any complications?

Let me tell you what happens when you swallow a burp or hold in a fart.

To hold in a fart, you would have to clench your anal sphincter muscles tight—you know the doors at the beginning and end of your anus. When you do this, you can successfully stop a fart from escaping, but inside your digestive tract, the pressure starts to build up.

You may start to feel pain or an uncomfortable bloating in your stomach that may be followed by the feeling of bubbles popping inside your tummy. The trapped gas then starts to make its way through your GI tract at which point you are going to start to feel the gas as a fluttery feeling in your belly followed by low gurgling noises.

Most of the trapped gas will remain thus, making its way around your GI tract, while some of it may seep into your bloodstream and find its way out when you exhale. Gas does not remain trapped forever, and will eventually make its way out as either a burp or a fart—unfortunately exploding, at times, as both.

Apart from the pain and discomfort you feel, holding in gas (fart) has not shown to be detrimental to your health, except that letting out a fart when needed can keep your digestive tract happy.

You can, of course, control gas buildup in your system by avoiding certain types of food that encourage the production of gas from your gut bacteria. Some of the food types that cause gas buildup include the following.

- Beans
- Cabbage, broccoli, and cauliflower
- Legumes
- Food that contains artificial sweeteners, especially xylitol and sorbitol.
- Beer
- Fizzy drinks

- Lactose which is a natural sugar present in milk and other dairy products.

Fructose which is a natural sugar that occurs in fruits, wheat, onions, and also bottled fruit drinks/soft drinks.

Try to limit high-protein diets and fatty food and see how you feel. If you notice you are less gassy after that, try to stick to that reduced ratio.

Also, dietary fibres, while essential for gut health, can cause excessive gas in some people. Try limiting food such as whole bread and whole grains and gauge the difference.

Other simple measures to adopt and avoid gas buildup is to eat and chew your food slowly to stop swallowing excess air. Make lifestyle changes such as quitting smoking, but do keep in mind that expelling gas is a natural phenomenon of your digestive cycle and should not be thought of otherwise.

3. Eat to Please Your Gut Bacteria

You can eat to please your gut bacteria by finding out about the types of bacterial microorganisms living in your intestinal microbiome. Learning about the types of bugs living in your GI tract makes it easy for you to manage the food you eat and work toward optimal health. By catering to the needs of the good bugs in your gut, you can help tip the scales in their favour by making sure you eat nothing to put that delicate balance out of sync and put yourself in danger of developing conditions such as dysbiosis.

You can eat to encourage your good bacteria by discovering the enterotype you belong to. And now, identifying your bacterial enterotype is simpler than you think, in fact, you can do the test at home. All you need is a microbiome testing kit.

The Microbiome Testing Kit

You can order these test kits online. They operate in much the same way a proper laboratory test is conducted where you need to add a sample of your poop to the provided container in the testing kit. The sample is then sent back to the company's lab for testing, which may take a few days or sometimes a week or more. It all depends on the company providing the home testing kits.

The types of results you get will again depend on the company you bought the kit from. But overall, they all test your stools to decipher the types of bacterial organisms living in your gut.

The levels of analysis are not as comprehensive as one that would be conducted at a lab where you can directly submit your stool sample, although the home-extracted sample is tested at a lab as well. Yet, online tests are not recognized as conclusive and should not be used to come to any sort of diagnosis or conclusion about your condition. That is something a healthcare provider must confirm after extensive and proper testing.

The home tests are a kind of preliminary analysis that tells you about the type of microorganisms in your gut and may include added results of any food sensitivities and inflammation triggers you may be dealing with. It serves the basic purpose of learning about the types of bacteria in your gut so you can start to eat right and please your intestinal microbiome.

Problems With Your Gut

Next, we are going to look at problems your GI tract encounters. Because your overall health starts in your gut.

You already learned about dysbiosis and the type of damage a gut microbiota that's out of sync can do because an unhealthy gut can impact various parts of your body. Therefore, it's important to be attuned to what's going on with your digestive tract in order to act in time to prevent any major diseases or conditions from taking place.

An unhealthy gut can be linked to numerous diseases, a fact that has been proven through research. Obesity, diabetes, rheumatoid arthritis, chronic fatigue, depression, mental health issues, and several autoimmune diseases are linked to problems with the gut (Vijay & Valdes, 2021).

What Is an Unhealthy Gut?

Digestive problems are almost always the first signs that tell you your gut is having problems. Maintaining the balance of your gut flora is of utmost importance and I have already explained the factors that lead to an imbalance of your good and bad bugs in your gut microbiome, that in turn cause the condition called dysbiosis.

Since your gut microbiome plays a major role in maintaining the health of your digestive system, conditions like dysbiosis that develop due to factors that cause harm to the good intestinal bacteria are pretty much the overall cause of problems in your entire GI tract.

You can prevent a lot of problems leading to the ill health of your gut microbiome, your gut barrier, and your digestive system as a whole, by paying close attention to the signals your body is sending you. Being attuned to when changes take place with you both physically and mentally are the essential signs to be able to seek help and an early diagnosis.

Symptoms that are linked to an unhealthy gut make diagnosing the problem easy. However, while some signs may be easy to detect, others are not. Listed below are the most common causes and reasons that lead to gut-related problems.

1. You Suddenly Develop a Sweet Tooth

This is almost a sneaky, little trick employed by the sugar-craving bad bacteria in your gut. When the balance goes off and your bad bacteria start to thrive, the micro-organisms will want food they crave, especially pathogenic bacteria. To ensure they receive their sugar cravings, these bacteria can influence your cravings by secreting a protein-peptide compound that is very similar to two hormones called leptin and ghrelin. Leptin controls your appetite and cravings while ghrelin controls your hunger pangs. So, you see the bacteria, which has a mind of its own is telling you, or rather manipulating you to eat their favourite food—sugar.

Solution: You need to re-establish your gut flora balance by increasing the number of good bugs there. Supplementing with probiotics will add more good bacteria to your gut microbiome while including prebiotics in your diet will help the good bacteria there to thrive and multiply.

Make every effort you can to support and help your good bacteria to multiply. Make a lifestyle change and consciously avoid eating too many sweet treats whenever you get the urge to feed your sweet cravings, try eating natural sugars such as greek yoghurt with berries, or dried fruit but also in moderation.

2. You Start to Experience More Than Normal Burping, Bloating, and Bad Breath

We already covered the effects of bacteria and how excessive production of gas was a by-product of bacteria digesting the food they consume. Lactose intolerance and food allergies happen when the quality of your gut microbiome is low. Since the diversity of bugs that thrive in your gut microbiome leads to a healthy cluster of gut flora, low-quality gut bacteria results in poor digestion and a lack of essential bacteria to break down compounds such as lactose (sugars found in dairy), and gluten. Gluten is a type of plant protein found in wheat, rye, barley and other grains. Gluten can trigger intolerance in some people, especially those with Celiac disease.

Such food that the bacteria in your gut cannot digest turns into 'trigger foods' for producing excessive gas and bloating. More on allergies and food intolerance later.

Bad breath is another complication of your gut microbiome going off balance. Halitosis develops for several reasons but mainly when the number of bad bacteria in your mouth starts to thrive.

This usually happens when the number of bacteria types that produce sulphur increases; to make matters worse, this type of bacteria lives on the tongue (one reason you must pay attention to brushing your tongue together with your teeth). The sulphur is released when the bacterial organisms start synthesising protein compounds in the food you eat; the result is the foul-smelling sulfuric gas that starts to emanate from the back of your tongue.

Solution: Concentrate on supplementing your digestive tract with beneficial compounds to boost your stomach acids. Drinking lemon water and apple cider vinegar mixed in a glass of water can help to balance the Ph levels of your stomach acids. If you constantly suffer from gas or feel bloated it would be wise to keep track of the food you eat, that way you will be able to easily backtrack and identify the food that often triggers the symptoms. Once you do avoid them and gauge the difference.

3. Diarrhoea, Gas, and Constipation

You know that your gut health can easily be measured by the quality of your poop. You know what to look for once you have pooped. But what happens if there is no poop to analyse because you are either constipated or passing very watery stools. Both are a sign your gut is having problems with the bugs that live there, which is most likely caused by an increase of bad bugs interfering with the proper digestive process.

Passing excessive gas or farting too much is a good indication that bad bacteria has taken over your gut microbiome. The result is poop that is out of the normal or missing totally. Do keep in mind that passing food faster than they are digested, which is what happens when you develop diarrhoea, is as equally bad as not passing stools at all since poop that remains in your digestive tract can become toxic and lead to several dire conditions.

Solution: Your diet plays a major role in avoiding constipation, diarrhoea, and gas; the first rule is to stay well-hydrated, supporting your intestinal mucosa which in turn makes it easy for the food to move along your gut. Include plenty of fibre-rich food to ensure you form healthy stools (more on fibre and food in the following chapters). Avoid too much caffeine and stress, which impacts the quality of your poop and increases stomach acidity that will also cause gas and burping. Ensure you avoid triggers that lead to dysbiosis.

4. Dealing With a Weak Immune System

Your gut has the power to influence almost 80% of your antibody secretion by sensitising your immune system to secrete antibodies whenever your internal system is at risk from outside infection. One of the main reasons your gut microbiome is so attuned to allergies and infections is its need to keep checking the food you eat is safe and not toxic to your system. Scientists are still not 100% sure about how the bacteria in your gut manage to influence your immune system, but letting your gut microbiome go off balance is a marker for your immune system to develop problems. Therefore, one sure sign that your gut is not up to its usual mark is when you keep dealing with infections constantly, or in short: when you keep getting sick on a more regular basis than before.

Solution: Support your gut microbiome to maintain your immune system. Avoid stressing out your system by ensuring you get adequate sleep, exercise, and rest. Eat plenty of gut-healthy food such as fermented types like kimchi. Ensure you eat a balanced diet consisting of all the right macro and micronutrients. Supplement on vitamin D by alternately getting loads of sunshine by making it a practice to indulge in morning walks, jogs or even dropping off the kids at school. Drink plenty of water and avoid too much caffeine. Enjoy a balanced lifestyle reducing stressors and decompressing at the end of the day by practising yoga or even mindfulness meditation (an online search will update you on how mindfulness meditation can be practised while going about your daily tasks).

Your gut-brain axis has a lot to do with changes in your mood and well-being which is why mood disorders can be linked to an unhealthy gut. Simply eating a balanced nutrition-dense diet is not enough if you are dealing with internal problems such as dysbiosis, leaky gut, and an imbalance of stomach acids.

Leaky gut syndrome will certainly deplete the number of nutrients your intestines can absorb from food before it filters through your damaged gut barrier. Likewise, an imbalance of your gut flora is going to interfere with the secretion of your feel-good hormones serotonin and dopamine. Therefore, it is not uncommon for people to be diagnosed with mental-health disorders, despite making efforts to eat balanced diets. They may be negligent in avoiding other factors that can cause dysbiosis such as leading sedentary lifestyles for example.

Solution: The only way to ensure your gut supports your mental health is to avoid the common and often stressed triggers that lead to gut damage like smoking, excessive alcohol consumption, etc. In addition, staying well-hydrated, and including plenty of gut-friendly food in your diet as well as supplementing with probiotics and digestive assist supplements are good practices to safeguard your mental health by keeping your gut happy.

5. Dealing With Skin Problems

If you want glowing healthy skin, ditch the expensive creams and start nurturing your gut because that's where healthy skin begins. Eczema and psoriasis are skin conditions linked to inflammation, leaky gut syndrome, and gut bacteria. Dry and flaky skin is often a sure sign your gut is unhealthy.

Since your skin helps your system to expel toxins, a malfunction in the process can cause the skin to suffer. The lymphatic system supports the expulsion of toxins and removing liquids from the intestines. Autoimmune diseases such as inflammation and leaky gut syndrome often cause a disruption to the lymphatic system. When this happens, proteins are not properly drained and will accumulate, causing swelling and blocks which try to push through your skin, which in turn will cause blisters, scaly skin, and red patches. Bad stomach bacteria can infect and cause disruptions and blocks in your lymphatic system.

Solution: Try to curb leaky gut syndrome and encourage the health of your gut lining. Bone broth is a good option to include in your diet for this purpose. Also, ensure you drink plenty of water and enjoy hot and cold showers alternatively. Plenty of exercise to help you sweat and keep your lymphatic system working as well as help your skin sweat out toxins will help. Get plenty of sunshine vitamin-D which is essential for the metabolism of calcium. Eat plenty of food rich in minerals, as well as vitamin A which is a fat-soluble vitamin. Omega 3 supplements will help to balance inflammation which is encouraged when your omega 3 supply goes off balance.

6. A Zap in Energy and Development of Poor Sleep Habits

Among the many hormones controlled by your gut-brain axis is melatonin. The hormone when secreted induces sleep. Light reduces its numbers which is why we wake up when it's daylight. But just like blue light that can interfere with your melatonin levels, your gut's ill health too can cause a disruption of its levels as melatonin is produced in your brain and gut.

Your microbiome impacts your sleep by influencing your circadian rhythm (CR) which is your natural sleep-wake cycle, as it controls melatonin and cortisol that influence that cycle. Because of the gut-brain connection, your gut influences your mood, and as you know an unhealthy gut can disrupt this, which in turn will have effects on the quality of your sleep; thus, affecting your melatonin and cortisol secretion. Conversely, poor sleep is going to affect the health of the bugs in your microbiome.

Cortisol, the alert hormone essential to complete your sleep-wake cycle when disrupted due to your gut health can impact how energised you feel during the day. Gut permeability which happens with leaky gut syndrome is a factor that affects the secretion of cortisol. A leaky gut affects the secretion of the hormone essential to keep you alert, energised, and stress free during the day.

A leaky gut can also cause a depletion of the number of nutrients your GI tract can absorb because so many filters out of your gut without getting digested. That too will contribute to depletion of energy levels, leaving you to deal with fatigue most of the time.

On an interesting note: There is research to suggest that the gut microbiome operates on its own 'microbial rhythm' that is similar to, and in tune with your natural circadian rhythm and is thus able to influence cognitive, metabolic, and immune functions while at the same time influencing your natural circadian rhythm too (Murakami & Tognini, 2020).

This connection keeps your bodily functions within a certain flow, and can at times even cause disruptions between the two. Research is still fairly new and ongoing as the vast gut microbiome and its full scope of functions is still a mystery to scientists.

7. Developing Food Allergies and Intolerances to Certain Types of Food

Allergies: The most common symptom of a food allergy is diarrhoea or bloating and gas because food allergies almost always develop in your gut.

Generally, food that does not agree with you and is left undigested and gets excreted as waste, which is basically your body rejecting and kicking out the foreign substances it does not like. However, developing conditions such as leaky gut can cause severe damage as it lets those toxic undigested food particles leak into your bloodstream causing your immune system to start fighting back.

The results of course are not pretty and can even lead to more serious food poisoning episodes. Common food types that are the usual suspects for causing food allergies are nuts, dairy, gluten, and plant food from the nightshade family that include eggplant, tomato, peppers and potato.

Intolerance: Developing an intolerance for a certain type of food is not classified as an allergy but simply means your body cannot tolerate those food types.

Sometimes with food intolerances, you may experience regurgitation of food, a few minutes after eating. This is an automatic reflex your digestive tract adopts at times to try and re-digest food particles that remain as a result of poor digestion.

Poor digestion is often due to an insufficiency of digestive enzymes needed to complete the task of breaking down carbs, fats, and proteins; dealing with insufficient enzymes to complete digestion is another feature identified as food intolerance. Citrus fruits, cabbage, and beans are common triggers of food intolerance. Gluten and dairy intolerance is quite often linked to leaky gut syndrome and is one of the markers to check for the condition. The reason is gut permeability which develops as a result; making your body react to certain types of food as toxins. Heightened immune reactions that lead to inflammation are associated with food sensitivities due to this reason. IBS too is a common denominator for someone developing food intolerances.

Most times it is hard to decipher between a food allergy and an intolerance. Because you will most likely experience similar symptoms, therefore, getting properly diagnosed by a healthcare provider is essential to start a proper course of treatment. You can of course do the home test to check your microbiome, as the first step toward getting a clue about what's going on with your gut, but is not a final diagnosis. Common symptoms of food allergies and intolerances include the following:

- Stomach cramps and pains

- Headaches or even migraines

- Sudden diarrhoea

- Excess Gas

- Suddenly developing the sniffles or a runny nose

A Look at Common Digestive Syndromes Related to Dysbiosis

Dysbiosis is associated with a number of diseases related to your digestive tract. Let's take a look at each one.

Coeliac Disease

Celiac/coeliac disease (CD) invades the small intestines and will change the environment of the gut microbiome. Dysbiosis is a marker for the disease which begins with the ingestion of gluten by people having a sensitivity or intolerance to the food substance. Since it alters the microbiome, CD is also associated with chronic inflammation.

A good indication that CD is on the rise among the modern population is the many gluten-free meals on offer at restaurants and as packaged food. Gluten can cause several problems for people having an intolerance to the substance but is particularly deadly for people dealing with CD.

While gluten on its own cannot destroy the gut, a combination of gluten and CD causes the immune system to go into overdrive, identifying the substance as an invasive toxin. The result is the immune system attacking the gut lining and making it permeable. In short, coeliac disease can cause holes in your intestines.

Symptoms of Celiac Disease

Some symptoms are caused by a lack of nutrients because as is the norm with dysbiosis, food particles leaking through the gut, prevent optimal absorption of the nutrients in them.

- Gas
- Nausea
- Bloating
- Abdominal pain
- Fatigue
- Diarrhoea
- Vomiting
- Headaches
- Anaemia
- Anxiety and depression
- Pain in the joints
- Dermatitis
- A tingling sensation in the feet and hands

What Causes Celiac Disease?

Recent findings show that bad gut bacteria are responsible for causing celiac disease. On analysing the gut microbiome of people dealing with CD, an imbalance of bacteria, where the good bacteria was reduced to make way for higher numbers of destructive bacteria was noted. Concluding that several bad bacteria species are responsible for the onset of the disease (Marasco et al., 2016).

Did you know that celiac disease was not known until the early 1900s?

Today, the disease can even affect infants between eight to twelve months and is widely spread. The main causes of the spread of CD are linked to our modern diets that are less diverse in terms of variety, are calorie-dense, low in nutrients, and are less fresh with processed and pre-packed foods taking precedence. An increase in caesarean births and widespread use of antibiotics are other contributing factors.

While the solution to the syndrome lies within your gut microbiome, your best course of action is to continue nurturing and nourishing your gut bacteria through healthy lifestyle habits and maintaining a gluten-free diet.

Crohn's Disease

This disease too is heavily linked to a shift in the gut microbiome, where bad bugs precede the number of good bugs. The disease is characterised by an inflammation of the intestines and is one of the conditions linked to inflammatory bowel disease (IBD); the other is ulcerative colitis.

Crohn's too is a modern disease and only started to appear in larger numbers around the 1950s. Symptoms include the following.

- Cramps
- Pain in the abdomen
- Diarrhoea
- Ulcers in the intestines

There is a genetic link to Crohn's which is linked to the immune system, however, it is not the only cause of the disease; dysbiosis remains a major marker for the development of Crohn's.

Research has revealed the presence of very specific types of bacteria in the gut microbiome of people dealing with Crohn's and it is suspected that due to the genetic link, the bacteria may be inherited (Hicklin, 2017).

Antibiotics, while being harmful to gut bacteria, seem to be more volatile among Crohn's patients. A simple lifestyle change to ensure your good gut bacteria remains healthy and strong to fight the invasive bugs is by far the best prevention for Crohn's.

Ulcerative Colitis

Affecting your large intestine, colon, and rectum, ulcerative colitis is the other condition linked to IBD. The main characteristics of the disease are ulcers and inflammation of the colon and rectum.

The disease has the potential to be life-threatening but while there still is no proper cure, timely diagnosis and treatment can help with controlling the symptoms. Ulcerative colitis is grouped according to where it occurs; thus, there are four types.

- Left-sided colitis—the inflammation, in this case, rises from the rectum up to the colon with symptoms ranging from diarrhoea with traces of blood, a feeling of wanting to pass stools urgently, cramps, and pain centred to the left side.

- Ulcerative proctitis—in this case, the inflammation occurs around the rectum with symptoms including bleeding at the site.
- Pancolitis—when this type of ulcerative colitis occurs, the entire length of the rectum gets affected and patients experience heavy bleeding with diarrhoea. Weight loss and fatigue take over together with cramps and bad abdominal pains.
- Proctosigmoiditis—the lower part of the colon and rectum are infected and inflamed. You may feel an urge to poop but find you are unable to have a bowel movement with this type. Bloody diarrhoea is commonly accompanied by cramps and pain in the abdomen.

The symptoms associated with ulcerative colitis include the following:

- Pain in the rectum
- Diarrhoea with traces of blood
- Cramps and pain in the stomach
- Fever
- Fatigue
- Stunted growth in children

Risk factors are attributed to a family history of the disease as well as dysbiosis since the disease is linked to the immune system attacking the body. Again, I will stress that a lifestyle change, and making smart choices in terms of your well-being are the best remedies to avoid or manage disease linked to IBD.

Inflammatory Bowel Syndrome (IBS)

One of the most common diseases affecting the lower gut, IBS, is a chronic disease that must be managed over time. Maintaining a healthy outlook on life is one of the most successful methods for managing IBS which can and is successfully managed by most people dealing with the syndrome.

Common symptoms include the following.

- A change in your pooping schedule is one of the first alerts
- Pain when passing stools, bloating or sudden abdominal cramps
- Your poop starts to look different from what you usually pass

While these symptoms are a common and broad range, you must seek medical help if you do develop any of these symptoms.

- Sudden vomiting
- You find it difficult to swallow
- Experience weight loss that is unaccountable
- Bleeding from the rectum
- A nagging pain in your abdomen that will not go away even when you pass gas
- You become anaemic

There is no specifically identified cause for IBS, however, the usual culprits are linked to a change in your gut microbiome, an increase of harmful gut bacteria, dealing with stress from a young age, poor intestinal muscle contractions that are not strong enough to properly push food along the gut as well as abnormalities in the immune system as is often caused by dysbiosis.

Maintain a healthy outlook toward your everyday life and avoid or manage the hassles of conditions like IBS, which rely on the ill-health of your gut to thrive.

How Does Your Gut Influence Your Weight?

Weight loss is a debatable subject for many, and indeed one that puts a lot of stress on your gut microbiome. Fad diets abound and many of us have been through a few, cutting carbs, and increasing proteins. Each time you do so, you are changing the environment of your gut flora.

Trying to keep up with society's image of 'perfection' is tough, which is why you must discard it as an unhealthy option. Having come this far, you know that weight and health management is more than paying attention to the number of calories you eat. You need to look at measures to keep your gut happy because just like your GI tract impacts all aspects of your wellbeing, your gut bacteria has a huge influence on your weight management.

Role of Gut Bacteria and Digestion for Weight Management

Your gut flora is diverse but it can be loosely grouped as the good guys and the bad guys. Your good bacteria manage your weight by impacting digestion and your metabolism; both are crucial for successful weight management.

To do this, you need to maintain a proper microbial balance in your gut. Too many bad bacteria reduce the diversity of your microbiome, and you know that proper digestion of all food types happens only when your gut bacteria is diverse. A healthy gut is one that has a diverse and thriving gut bacteria that is essentially made up of good bugs.

Without proper diversity of gut bacteria, your GI tract will not be able to break down all food types, and when that happens, you are looking at poor metabolization of nutrients and greater storage of undigested calories as fat.

Gut Bacteria, Hormone Management, and Weight Gain

Problems that arise when your gut bacteria interferes with the proper secretion of hormones can impact your weight management. This is a greater problem for women when the expulsion of oestrogen is hindered.

Oestrogen, once used, must be expelled from the body with your poop. However, if your bad gut bacteria increases, you are at risk of some of that bad bacteria influencing the reabsorption of used oestrogen. The hormone is reabsorbed and gets stored in your liver until it is expelled by the organ as a toxin. However, if on top of your gut bacteria losing its diversity your liver function too is hindered (causes being too much alcohol, and caffeine), your liver cannot expel the oestrogen which then gets deposited in your fat cells mostly on the arms, hips and thighs.

How to Support Your Gut Bacteria For Optimal Weight Management

- Encourage the secretion of hydrochloric acid in your stomach by drinking water with lemon juice or apple cider vinegar first thing in the morning on an empty stomach.

- Choose nutrition-dense food to stay energised.

- Feed your gut microbiome with prebiotics and fermented food.

- Encourage good digestion with fibre-rich meals.

- Eat slowly and chew your food thoroughly to further support proper digestion.

Now that you know more about your gut and keeping it healthy, you must learn about listening to your gut and understanding the signals and messages it's sending your way. What is *your* gut telling you?

Chapter 3:
You and Your Gut—A Unique Relationship

Let's look at tuning into your gut; taking that 'gut feeling' more seriously and learning to stop and pay attention to the needs of your most important biological system.

As you know, we all possess a highly diverse gut microbiome, and catering to its needs is beneficial for overall well-being. To initiate the change, you must become aware of your gut's unique needs because what works for your friend may turn out to be toxic for you. Awareness and being in tune with your gut is also the first step toward changing your lifestyle.

In this chapter, we will look at techniques and methods you can use to monitor your gut and track any important changes that take place. Using your five senses is essential to becoming sensitive to what your gut is telling you and for deciphering the messages.

Your gut is one of the smartest systems you possess and when you learn to listen to what it's telling you, you will be able to discover a whole range of unique characteristics about yourself.

Your gut in turn is sensitive to all your needs and watches out for your well-being by sending you warning signals when all is not okay; picking up on those signals in a timely manner will save you a whole lot of health risks in the long run.

Your gut sends you messages using all your receptors.

- Sight

- Sound
- Smell
- Taste
- Feel

Let's look at tuning into these senses and heightening your awareness of what these receptors are picking up. I will also introduce you to the concept of maintaining a food journal. It will be an invaluable tool for managing your gut health and becoming aware of triggers that cause your system distress.

Are You Listening to Your Gut?

Your gut has been talking to you all along, communicating to let you know when all is not well and problems are on the horizon. You probably didn't realise this, and you may have overlooked some very important messages along the way. Listening to your gut is not some complicated task that requires you to get qualified in some special language. It's your gut after all, and it's watching out for your wellbeing.

Let's look at how you can get to know more about your gut and become alert to all warning signals being sent your way using your five senses.

Sight—This one is for your poop. We already discussed the importance of examining your poop and using the Bristol Stool Chart to evaluate its appearance. You know you can tell a lot about the health of your gut from the shape, size and texture of your poop. Apart from those already explored, watch out for dark reddish, blackish or tarry-looking poop which can quite often be due to internal bleeding in your intestines or stomach.

If you have any concerns or something doesn't seem normal, then speak to your healthcare provider.

Sound—Your stomach growling or gurgling could mean different things. The commonest reason is the digestion process that is taking place. Digestive juices, food and gas getting pushed through your intestines during the digestion process can be noisy, with no way to mask the noises. Luckily, they are not too loud and cannot be heard quite as distinctly as when your stomach growls to say it is empty. Your stomach growling to indicate hunger is due to the secretion of ghrelin, the hunger hormone which too is produced in the gut.

Smell—Farts tell you a lot about your microbiome and the food you have eaten. Some foods, such as sugars, are lapped up by the bad bacteria in your gut to produce gases that escape as farts. Others like high-protein meals are metabolised by gut bacteria which produce a foul-smelling sulfuric gas—the answer to those rotten-eggy-smelling farts! Of course, it's a natural phenomenon to eat food that contains protein compounds.

Any change in smells must be duly noted because the smell of farts, burps and gas expelled from your body can also tell you if the food you ate is left undigested, and whether you are under too much stress.

Feel—Abdominal pains can be related to several digestive syndromes such as IBS and IBD for example. Abdominal pains can also occur as a result of your digestive process where your gut contracts to push food along your intestines. Bloating too happens because of gas produced from something you ate and can cause pain. Gallstones obstructing your bile duct can induce pain too as do the ulcerations and swelling of the intestines caused by Crohn's disease.

Taste—you know your food is being brought up by the strong acidic taste you feel in your mouth. It's due to a mixture of stomach acids and undigested food that is being regurgitated by your digestive tract in a bid to try and redigest it. This could mean several things; your gut microbiome is not diverse enough to digest the food, you have an intolerance to that type of food or you are dealing with a lack of digestive enzymes needed to complete the process.

Assessing the Health of Your Gut

Not all signals and signs can be picked up easily, and if you suspect you may be dealing with a gut-related problem, the digestive health assessment test listed here has been put together by top gut-health experts to help you to make an evaluation of your digestive health based on symptoms and lifestyle habits. It will help you to better understand if you must seek medical help or not.

Gut Health Assessment

Section A	Yes ✓	No ✓
There is a consistent change in my bowel-movement schedule, and it cannot be due to medication, a change in my diet or stress.		
There have been traces of blood in my poop		
I am dealing with persistent pain in my stomach		

and it's not due to stress or a change in my diet.		
I am experiencing sudden weight loss which is unexplainable (over 24 kg/4 lbs)		
I have an unexplained loss of appetite and I feel unwell quite often but I don't know why.		
I am experiencing a continuously upset gut, and simply feel unwell with symptoms of sweating, shivering and fever		
Having a YES answer to even one of the questions in section A is an indication of a gastrointestinal problem that needs to be analysed by a healthcare provider.		
Section B		
I need to poop many times a day, or I am dealing with constipation.		
My stools are sometimes hard pellets or soft and runny.		
Although I feel the need to pass stools, I actually cannot.		
My stomach acts up every time I deal with stress		
I have several food sensitivities/allergies		

Together with bowel or abdominal problems, I experience fatigue, and muscle pains and also deal with indigestion on a regular basis.		
My stomach is very sensitive and always giving me trouble, it's making me very depressed.		
I deal with severe bloating and it makes me look obese.		
If you answered YES to any of these questions but NO to those in section A it is likely you have a milder gut problem like IBS		
Section C		
I often skip breakfast		
I very rarely eat cereal for breakfast, and I do not load up on five fruits and vegetables a day.		
Exercise is not a regular habit for me.		
I am in the habit of watching television for at least two hours a day.		
I enjoy an alcoholic drink almost daily		
I have gained weight		

I am a regular smoker		
I deal with a lot of stress		
My sleep quality and quota are low		
Answering YES to even one of the questions in this section suggests you need to make a serious lifestyle change in view of your wellbeing.		

This guide is merely an assessment help and does not offer a conclusive diagnosis of any condition. If you do suspect you may be dealing with gut-related conditions, seeking medical help at your earliest convenience is the best solution.

Start Journaling Your Gut Changes

Record your digestive changes by keeping a food and poop journal and you will be able to successfully monitor any changes that take place in your digestive tract.

You know the days you simply feel off and try to recall what it was you did or ate the previous few days to make you feel this way?

Or the times you feel really energised and ready to take on the world?

Those changes in your behaviour and overall health that you can easily link to what you ate. And by keeping the poop journal, you can easily backtrack to identify when the change started to reflect in your stools. There are several ways to maintain a journal. You can do it the old-fashioned way by going out and getting yourself a handy little journal that fits right in your purse, backpack or pocket. One that you can take along to record every titbit you eat. Or you can choose to download an app that serves the purpose just as well.

There are several well-received journaling apps you can download to your smartphone to make the entire process smooth, easy and digitised. Because when using an app for journaling, you can do so much more. You can sync your work between devices, add reminders, combine your data for analysis, and even export information the moment you find a better app. Here is a list of the top journaling apps in the market.

- Penzu—this app works across Android, iOS, and web applications and is one of those high-tech gadgets that have an old-fashioned feel. You can use WordPress to add your entries which work on a very user-friendly WYSIWYG (what you see is what you get) platform.

- Day One—works on Mac, iOS, Android, and WatchOS. The app is one of the more popular ones, and is loved for its variety of features and ease of use as well as the attractive templates which make journaling a pleasure.

- Memento—runs on the iOS system. Memento is kind of like your own private Facebook, Twitter, Instagram, and other platforms, all rolled into one. The app combines all your social media updates onto one platform to keep you informed of where you were and what you did. It is perfect for keeping track of your social life for starters and remembering where you may have over-indulged or accidentally eaten food your gut cannot tolerate.

- Dabble Me—is a web journal that works with your email to ensure you receive a daily reminder to update your journal. If you love writing long notes to yourself, this is the app for you, Dabble Me is user-friendly and can be easily accessed over the web.

These are just a few of the journal apps out there, a quick online search will easily help you decide on which one to start using. Of course, if you are more of an old-fashioned person you will find several sample journal pages you can print, a good place to start is Pinterest.

Food Journal

A food journal is ideal if you are constantly dealing with allergies, and food intolerances. Keeping a record of everything you eat or drink for a minimum of one week will help you to discover a few truths about food types your body is capable of handling. Make sure you take your journal along with you wherever you go unless, of course, it's an app you carry on your smartphone.

Here are some samples of the type of data you need to include in your food journal.

What You Ate

- List every type of food you ate and try to be very specific about everything that was included in each meal.
- Add in the extras; sauces, toppings, spices, condiments, dressings, and other extras.

- Try to add quantity where possible. Such as how many crackers you ate, or how many sashimi rolls you enjoyed. Try to add weight and volume measurements as best you can. For example half a cup of rice, and an ounce of salad dressing. It may be difficult, especially when you eat out, but do your best and try adding rough quantities.

When You Ate, Where You ate, With What You Ate, With Who You Ate, and What You Were Doing at the Time

- Add in the time of day you ate (lunch, tea, or an afternoon snack)
- Where you ate the meal. At work, school, home, or a friend's house?
- What did you have your meal with? If you are on any medication at the time, include that, a glass of wine, or anything else you may have paired the meal with.
- Who you ate the meal with. A friend, colleagues from work, family, and so on.
- What you were doing at the time of eating the meal. Watching television, you were at the game enjoying the hotdog, or you were gaming and enjoying a snack.

Symptoms You Experienced After the Meal

- Go ahead and list every one of the symptoms you experienced. Even if it is the standard gas, bloating, and burping.
- List the standard non-dramatic ones too like nausea, vomiting, and diarrhoea.

- Have a good think and be observant, there may be more subtle symptoms you overlook such as joint pain you get after a meal, an elevation in your stress levels or even suddenly going blank as in losing your memory. Due to the gut-brain axis, there are some foods that contribute to the inflammatory process to impair both learning abilities and memory retention. Such foods include unhealthy industrial seed oils, simple/refined carbs, and high-sugar meals.

- Use a scale of 1–10 to define how severe the symptoms were, how bad you felt and for how long they lasted.

- Use your journal entries to shift back and make connections with symptoms that decide to show up a few days after you've eaten a certain meal. If you can't link a certain symptom to your present situation, chances are its roots are in something you ate, or a combination of what you ingested that's causing you discomfort at a later stage.

What Your Mood Was at the Time of Eating the Meal

- Were you happy, sad, angry, bored, or stressed. Mood is a huge influencer on appetite, and can equally impact symptoms you experience after. For example, stress can make you seek food that is high in sugar and fat. What we like to call comfort food is often a need to eat a certain type of food triggered by an emotion.

Exercise Levels

- Jot down how active you were on that day. Did you exercise? Or did you binge-watch television for two hours? If you did exercise, make sure you enter how long you did and the intensity of the workout.

Bowel Movements

- Enter the time you had a bowel movement for the day.
- Have a look at and write down the type of poop you passed. You can refer to the Bristol Stool Chart for ease.

The Days Sleep Schedule

- Did you enjoy a restful sleep, or were you tossing and turning all night long dealing with stomach cramps?

Try the Elimination Diet Technique to Identify Food Intolerances

Apart from your journal, you can use the elimination-diet technique to identify trigger foods that are causing your inflammation and other food sensitivity issues. Taking out the trigger foods from your diet should be controlled for at least a month to properly gauge their impact on your gut once you reintroduce them to your diet.

Elimination diets are not to be tried when you feel something is off, taking time to practice one and get to know your gut tolerances and intolerances will save you a lot of surprise trouble.

The standard 'watch out' for symptoms is inflammation which is basically the leading cause for most gut problems as well as other chronic diseases such as arthritis and even cancers.

Elimination diets can be conducted in several ways; some are pretty basic and ideal if you are not really suffering from any allergies or food intolerances. Others can be very specific if you suspect an intolerance to a specific type of food.

Here are some of the more popular elimination diets

- Full-elimination diet—a full elimination means you take out all food types identified as a cause for an intolerance. Included are nightshade plant varieties, citrus fruits, starches as well food containing gluten, nut, and seeds, legumes, dairy, meat and fish, eggs, fats including butter, margarine and shortening (hydrogenated oils which are vegetable seed oils that have been chemically altered to stay solid at room temperature), spreads and mayonnaise, liquids such as tea, coffee, sodas, alcohol and others containing caffeine, sugars, and artificial sweeteners.

- Basic elimination—on the basic-elimination diet you take out one or two of the suspected food groups. Let's say you are lactose intolerant, then you eliminate dairy and all dairy products, or if you have an intolerance to gluten you keep out starches and other gluten-containing food products. Alcohol too is stopped during this time.

- Elimination of carbohydrates (the Ketogenic diet)—take out carbs, essentially refined grains, simple carbs, and sugars

- The FODMAP-elimination diet—FODMAP stands for fermentable oligosaccharides, disaccharides, monosaccharides, and polyols. These are short-chain carbohydrates your body finds tough to digest. This elimination diet is generally conducted in three stages and is aimed at reducing IBS. A lot of processed foods and ready-to-eat meals generally fall into the FODMAP category.

- Nightshade elimination—taking out food that belongs to the nightshade family is how this diet works. While becoming intolerant to some people, vegetables that belong to the nightshade family contain several essential nutrients, therefore the normal practice is to replace these with alternates that are similarly nutritious.

  Choose sweet potatoes instead of white potatoes, opt for more citrus fruits to make up for the loss of vitamin C contained in most nightshades, add more dark green leafy vegetables such as kale and spinach to bump up your vitamins, minerals, and fibre.

- The paleo diet—following this way of eating will require you to stick to the basics just like your hunter-gatherer ancestors. Your gut is probably most adapted to this type of eating instead of having to adapt to the metabolization of many modern foods. On the paleo eating plan, you stick to fish and lean meats, fruits, vegetables, and nuts.

Seeking medical help before you begin an elimination diet will ensure you follow the proper steps that will safeguard your wellbeing. A nutritionist or healthcare provider will be able to advise you on the practicality, healthwise, of eliminating certain foods from your diet for an extended period. Plus, they may advise you on what type of food intolerance you may be suffering from based on your symptoms, thus making it easy for you to decide on the type of elimination diet to follow.

Easy Elimination Diet to Try at Home

If you want to keep your experiment simple, you can try this easy elimination diet at home, to get a rough indication of any food types you may be intolerant of, the easy step-by-step process will help you to explore and experiment.

Step 1:

Gauge your symptoms. First, you must make a list of your symptoms so you can decide on the type of elimination path you must follow. Make a list of potential signs you have a food intolerance.

- Skin sensitivities
- Bloating
- Gas
- Constipation that's intermittent
- Sudden allergies
- Fuzzy brain where you seem to suddenly forget things
- Mood changes

Once you start evaluating your situation, you are going to notice some of these symptoms you did not before, and they are going to be very enlightening on getting started with a rough assessment of your condition.

Step 2:

Start your elimination process. The general norm is to use a 23-day period to eliminate food types you suspect are causing your gut problems. Start the basic-elimination diet on step 2, where you take out antibiotics, and alcohol together with the most likely food group causing your intolerance.

Why must I follow the eating plan for 23 days?

It takes at least 21 days for reactive proteins produced as a result of your immune system reacting to foreign particles, to filter out, therefore, stopping foods you suspect of causing an immune reaction. This time frame will help you to make a proper assessment of your symptoms and any improvements that take place once the foods are eliminated.

Why must I eliminate alcohol?

High in sugars, alcohol feeds your bad gut bacteria. Simply eliminating food containing yeast will not be enough if you continue to consume alcohol as alcohol encourages yeast to multiply in your intestines. Taking out booze for 21–23 days will give you a chance to experience a biological reset where you start to feel healthier and less anxious because alcohol can increase your stress levels by influencing the release of more cortisol and interferes with parts of the brain that manage mood and curtails stress levels (Anthenelli & Grandison, 2012).

Basic Elimination Chart for Two Weeks or 4 Weeks

2 Week Diet Plan	4 Week Diet Plan	Steps to Follow
Day 1	Day-1	Start your elimination diet
Day 2–7	2 to 7 days	Symptoms are more pronounced on days 1 and 2
Day 8–17	Day 8–30	Symptoms start to diminish once the foodstuff causing the intolerance is eliminated.

Step 3:

Time to go shopping. Once you have done your symptom analysis and drawn up your food-elimination list, you can put together a grocery list. You will be surprised to see that despite the elimination process you can still go grocery shopping and look forward to putting together some interesting meal options.

What should I shop for?

- Meats and fish 30%—try to eat as clean as possible by eliminating possible pollutants.

  Choose—grass-fed, organic, free range, antibiotic-free, hormone-free meats, and fish. Opt for lean beef, chicken breasts, and wild-caught fish over farm-bred varieties. Eat plenty of fatty fish like sardine, salmon, cod, halibut, and herring.

- Plant food 70%—includes any type of vegetables and fruits, nuts, sweet potato, and grains that are gluten-free (gluten-free oats, quinoa, buckwheat, brown rice, corn), plant-based fats choose healthy oils like avocado, coconut, flax seed, walnut, and extra virgin olive oil.

- Salt and spices.

- Eat fresh, include plenty of salads and dietary fibres; try to make your meals at home. Even simple basic recipes will do as long as you avoid eating food cooked outside of your home as much as possible, as they may contain traces of ingredients you are trying to eliminate.

- You can try meal-kit delivery services in your neighbourhood for pre-cut, measured and neatly-packed ingredients, all you do is put the recipe together. They are great if you are busy and will cater to your choice of diet making sure you don't eat any of the eliminated food items. A simple online search will help you to locate the best meal kit delivery service closest to your home.

What to Avoid:

- Fish containing high levels of mercury and farm-bred fish. Avoid sharks, barramundi, swordfish, southern bluefin tuna, and orange roughy.

- Processed health bars, most contain added sugars. You can make your own protein bars at home. There are plenty of easy recipes online or choose the organic low sugar varieties.

- Limit carbs even if they are gluten-free, such as gluten-free bread. While these are alright to eat during your elimination diet, they are not good in excessive quantities.

Step 4:

After the 23 days have passed and you have recorded the changes you have observed, it's time to start reintroducing some of the eliminated foods back into your diet. However, this does not mean you start eating all of the eliminated food at once; you start by reintroducing one of the eliminated foods.

How do I start reintroducing the food?

Let's say you take one eliminated item—eggs. You then eat eggs on day 24. Observe to make sure there are no symptoms by waiting for 48 hours. You then reintroduce the same food back to your diet once more and observe your body's reaction. If there are no symptoms to cause you alarm, decide on continuing to eat the food. You may then move on to reintroducing the next item of food and follow the same procedure.

Step 5:

Listen to your body. Once you start your 21–23-day elimination diet, you are going to start feeling the effects of cutting out certain types of food. There will be a few positive changes you will observe along the way.

- Your skin allergy may clear up.
- Your body will no longer be bloated.
- Frequent flatulence and gassy feelings may subside.
- You may feel more energised.
- More alert with brain fog clearing up.

Use your journal to record all these changes as well as the foods you are avoiding and those you are eating. The elimination process will help you to pinpoint how each food type reacts with your gut. If you no longer suffer from bloating and gas, but find the symptoms have returned as soon as you eat gluten again, you know what the culprit is. It's no complicated process and is in fact one of the easiest methods to find out about your food reactions which a blood test is incapable of doing.

Read the Food Value Labels of All Food You Buy

One sure way to spot hidden ingredients that can easily trigger your intolerances is to read the food value labels.

For example, avoiding dairy means you have to be careful about not eating custard, milk chocolate, whey, casein, pudding, and other dairy containing foods. The only way to spot the hidden ingredients is to read the labels. Or make your meals from scratch at home.

Make Sure You Are Ready

When starting an elimination diet, it's important to make sure you are in a position to do so. Consider the disturbances and whether you are in a position to take on the challenge. Are you financially able to make the changes to your diet, to stock up on new ingredients?

Do you have the time to cook alternate meals and monitor your symptoms?

Only start when you are in a position to make a 100% commitment thereby ensuring the success and accuracy of the entire experiment.

Maintaining a Poop Journal—What Must You Include

Yes, there is such a thing and it is indeed a very handy method to keep track of your gut health because poop as I said, is your guts, exterior representative.

If you constantly suffer from irregular bowel movements, it's important to keep track of your poop cycles to get a better understanding of when you pooped, and why it looks the way it does. It will assist you to answer simple questions that will help you to judge the health of your gut, as well as, keep track of your lifestyle habits that impact your gut.

Enter every bowel movement you have in your journal and you can easily backtrack whenever trouble starts to brew with your gut. Here are some points to add to your poop journal so you can easily track your poop changes.

- Log in the appearance of your poop. Refer to the Bristol Stool Chart and use the number guide as a reference to mark the type of poop you see in the bowl by colour, and size.

- How long did you take to poop. Make a note of this every time you pass stools. And note down how much you had to strain, if at all, and how you felt once you finally passed the stools—did you feel empty?

    On average, a person takes about 12 seconds to pass stools, but at times it takes longer so you may add a buffer of no more than 10 minutes tops for all the time you spend in the loo.

    Once you poop, avoid hanging around in there, (no matter how much you like the privacy) If you habitually sit for too long on a toilet you will put additional strain on your rectum and anus. Since your rectum is hanging inside the toilet bowl, blood gets drawn to the vessels there and can at times cause clots that are aggravated by extra pressure from you straining to pass stools; the result is quite often haemorrhoids. Also called piles, haemorrhoids are blocked, bulgy veins that appear in the rectum.

Try to jot down a measure of how much you had to strain to pass the poop, use a scale of 1–10, associating pain, from moderate to high if you felt any for the higher numbers on the scale.

Sometimes passing dry, very large stools, is an added strain, where you sometimes feel pain as it passes through your rectum. The reason is often due to an insufficient intake of fluids. You will be able to compare these occasions with your food journal where you can compare your diet against the poop to notice significant influences between the two.

- Check for particles of undigested food in your poop, and look out for excess mucus and possibly traces of blood.

Why do I see these in my poop?

First, check on what you ate, we already covered the type of food that causes colour changes in stools, rule out those possibilities.

Bacterial infections in the gut are often the cause of excess mucus in the stools while Crohn's and ulcerative colitis are possible causes for blood and mucus to appear in your poop, only a proper medical evaluation will give you a correct diagnosis which you can get in a timely manner by paying attention to and detecting such changes in your poop.

- Make a note of your stress levels. Use a variable scale of 1–10 to measure your mood and stress levels with 10 being the highest.

- Did you exercise? If you did record the workout and for how long. Exercise can be any form of physical activity you enjoy, and will include walking, dancing, or other forms of activity you may enjoy as a way to stay active.

And to prove just how important a poop diary is, let me introduce you to the top five poop apps designed specially to help you keep a track of your poop and analyse everything else you did in between.

1. PoopLog

Designed for the Android system the PoopLog app lets you keep track of your stools by using the Bristol Stool Chart.

2. Bowel Movement Pro

Designed for the iOS system. With this app, you can track the number of times you passed stools and also let you log in its texture.

3. Poop Diary

Aren't you just loving these names?

Poop Diary not only tracks your bowel movements but is smart enough to offer you statistics to better analyse your situation like times when you were constipated.

4. Places I've Pooped

This app is for your poop to check-in. A kind 'poop was there' app that lets you keep a track of all the places you pooped.

5. PoopMD

This app offers a diagnostic feature that lets you analyse your poop against potential life-threatening conditions such as biliary atresia, a liver disease.

The Transit Time Test

What does the transit time test do?

Gut transit time refers to how long the food you ate takes to transition through the digestive process, running along your GI tract to finally be expelled as poop. In short, it is the time between when you ate breakfast to the next poop.

The gut transition time is seen as an important link for determining the health of your gut microbiome and the entire digestive process.

What is the ideal transition time?

- 12 to 48 hours is considered a healthy transition time allowing your digestive tract enough time to properly metabolise and absorb all the nutrients from the food you ate. There are of course variations to this time that generally indicate that your GI tract may be having problems.

A Too Fast Transition Time

If you have a poop within 10 hours of eating a meal it's an indication the food moved too fast through your digestive tract.

When food moves it is not sitting in your intestines and stomach long enough to get properly broken down or for the nutrients to be absorbed. You are basically pooping out food that has not had time to be properly digested and absorbed.

What are the risks?

- You can develop a nutrient deficiency.

- It's an indication that digestive enzymes are in low supply and you could be at risk from celiac disease, Crohn's disease, ulcerative colitis and IBS.

A Too Slow Transition Time

If you poop about 72 hours after eating a meal it is a sure sign of constipation. The food to poop transition taking place after such a long duration is a signal that you need to check for the following markers.

- Dysbiosis. A gut flora imbalance.

- Bloating and gas

- Toxins that may have built up in your gut as a result of various diseases, and also leaky gut syndrome making your intestines permeable.

- SIBO

How Can I Test My Transit Time?

A professionally conducted transit time test will consist of you swallowing a small pill that has a transmitter attached to it. The unit sends data to a portable receiver you will wear. Your healthcare provider will then use this data to analyse how smoothly your GI tract is functioning. Another option is swallowing a dye capsule that, once leaked, can be tracked as the dye progresses through your GI tract.

Apart from these professionally conducted tests, there is a simple cost-free test you can do at home.

At Home Bowel Transit Test

Choose a food marker, which is something you can eat, that will show in your poop. Try any one of the following markers.

- Two teaspoons of white sesame seeds. You may mix it in a glass of water.
- A cup of beetroot cooked or raw
- A cup of sweetcorn

Once you plan the bowel transit test date, avoid eating any of the marker food you choose for at least a week.

Start the Test

- On the day of the test eat the marker food an hour before the meal you choose to do the test with. Make a note of the time and the date.
- Watch out for signs of the marker food in your poop, make a note of the first time you spot it and write down the time and date.
- Calculate your bowel transit time by checking for the difference between the time you ate the marker food to the first time you saw it in your poop.

Check your poop transit time and compare it against the ideal transition time of 12 to 48 hours from which you can make an initial diagnosis and decide on further investigations.

The Aim For 30 Test

You know the *five fruits and veg a day* rule, but do you know about the amazing effects the 30 plant foods a week have on your gut microbiome?

It's pretty awesome and has been scientifically proven to have a very beneficial effect on your gut microbiome.

Testing was conducted by the American Gut Project where 10,000 scientists based across the globe were selected and then tested for gut microbiome diversity (McDonald et al., 2018).

Stool samples obtained from the scientists showed a very significant difference in gut bacteria based on the diets of each individual. Those who ate a mix of over 30 different plant foods a week had a healthy and very diverse mix of gut bacteria in comparison to the individuals who ate 10 or less.

Those who included more than 30 plant foods in their diets tested for higher levels of short chain fatty acids that offer a range of benefits to the gut starting with strengthening the intestinal walls.

What Can I Include to Make Up My 30 Plant Foods a Week?

Quite a lot actually. Because plant food is not merely fruits and vegetables; the range is quite diverse.

Types of Plant Food

- Fruits
- Legumes
- Vegetables
- Pulses
- Nuts
- Seeds
- Herbs
- Spices
- Cereals

Remember that the more colour you add to your diet the broader your nutritional intake will be.

What Can I Eat for a Week?

Here is a list of plant food you can use to make sure you include plenty of variety and numbers in your diet from every type. Don't be afraid to experiment and try types of plant food you have never eaten before. There are plenty of easy online recipes out there that make it easy to throw a delicious meal together with basic ingredients. And when it comes to vegetarian or vegan options the choices are endless and very taste-centric.

Sample Plant Food to Choose For Weekly Meal Planning

1. **Vegetables**
    - Onion (red, white, yellow, or spring)
    - Peppers (red, yellow, green, orange)
    - Garlic
    - Broccoli
    - Potatoes (sweet, red, white, baby)
    - Leafy greens (kale, spinach)
    - Brussels sprouts
    - Cauliflower
2. **Fruits**
    - Banana
    - Apples
    - Pear
    - Avocado
    - Blueberries
    - Citrus (lemon, orange, lime, satsuma)
    - Seasonal fruits
    - Kiwi
    - Raspberry
3. **Legumes and pulses**
    - Chickpeas
    - Lentils

- Kidney beans
- Black beans
- Soya

4. **Cereals**
   - Oats (preferably gluten-free)
   - Brown rice
   - Bran flakes
   - Muesli

5. **Herbs and spices**
   - Turmeric
   - Ginger
   - Cumin
   - Oregano

6. **Nuts and Seeds**
   - Walnuts
   - Mixed seeds

7. **Other important additions**
   - Plant-based milks that do not contain any stabilisers or preservatives
   - Olive oil
   - Live coconut yoghurt
   - Sauerkraut
   - Kimchi
   - Kombucha

Tips to Easily Include Plant Foods in Your Diet

Go ahead and meet that 30-a-week challenge with gusto. Your gut is going to love it and so will you once you start to experience the positive changes.

Meal Plan

Start meal planning. This means you must be organised and avoid visiting the supermarket to pick up stuff randomly, such trips often end up with impulse purchases, and when it comes to food, you often end up taking home an array of unhealthy processed foods.

Instead, check for vegetarian recipes online. Once you choose a few, decide on your week's meals and go ahead and make up a list. A list is a marvellous tool to keep you on track at the supermarket. Consider making up a weekly shopping list you can cover over a weekend and manage your busy weekday meals easily.

Maintain Your Food Journal

A food journal will be highly beneficial once you start your *30-a-week* challenge and you increase the variety to your diet. The journal will help you to backtrack and check on what you ate whenever the need arises. It is also an excellent method to eliminate or accept certain plant food types based on your guts reaction to each type.

Change Your Standard Meal Types

There is no hard and fast rule to say you must continue to eat your plant-based meal according to your standard cooking methods or recipes. Change up the ingredients and you will discover some very pleasant flavour combinations you will want to add to your permanent collection of recipes. Here are a few ideas for changing up your meal plans.

- Choose to eat the same vegetable in different types such as potatoes which have several different varieties.

- Choose vegetarian pasta delights. Forget the meat, and load your pasta with some nutrition-packed veggies, and your gut and tastebuds will love it. Have you tried pasta with peas, spinach, red beans, chickpeas, and even lentils? It's the perfect comfort food that is delicious and good for you.

- Choose the same veg in a rainbow of colours. Onions, cabbage, and peppers are fine examples. You are not required to stick to just red peppers or white onions all the time. Go ahead and experiment and discover a whole range of new flavours.

- Make your own portion of mixed nuts. A bag of almonds can be made so much more interesting and nutritious with a few additions. A handful of Brazil nuts, hazel nuts, walnuts, and sunflower seeds will be good little ingredients to have at home. Use them to dress up your cereal or salads and enjoy the crunch as well as a variety of tastes.

- Choose mixed salads instead of singles. There are plenty of pre-packed salad mixes that include mixed leaves for you to enjoy. Even if you think certain leaves or vegetables may not taste right, trying something different is definitely going to be a pleasant experience.

Go for Fermented Veggies

One of the best ways to preserve food and also make it gut healthy is to ferment it. You can have a lovely ready-to-eat side any time you fancy a taste by choosing to make a couple of jars of your favourite fermented plant foods.

Check out the recipes for kimchi which can be made with a variety of vegetables and then popped in the refrigerator to enjoy whenever you feel the need. Other types of fermented plant food options you can make at home and keep in the refrigerator include the following.

- Pickled garlic
- Olives
- Sauerkraut

All fermented food is gut-friendly and helps the good bugs in your microbiome thrive. Lactic acid bacteria that help to ferment sugars are very beneficial to your gut microbiome and are one of the essential good bugs that you can add to your microbiome as probiotics through fermented foods. Check out the recipes online for making your own fermented treats to be stored in jars and placed in the refrigerator.

Go Ahead and Freeze

Frozen food is just as nutritious as fresh food. Therefore, I highly recommend you use your freezer and fridge to store your week's grocery shopping. Vegetables, fruits, and berries can be frozen and used in many meals without compromising their food values.

- Frozen berries, fruits, and leafy greens like spinach and kale can be easily added to smoothies and soups.
- Frozen corn kernels, diced carrots, peas, and other cooked and frozen grains can be used to make quick stir-fries with no compromise on flavour.
- You can even chop up the ingredients for a vegetable soup—carrots, potato, celery, onions, and others and freeze them together. Simply add a lot to the recipe when you are making it, even top it up with ham, bacon, chicken, or any other meat of your choice if you decide to make it a non-veg meal.

Star Ingredients That are Very Gut-Friendly

Just like you have your favourite type of foods, your good gut bacteria have theirs. Listed here are top superfoods that are gut-friendly, and packed with essential nutrients while being absolutely delicious.

Having these ingredients in stock at home will make healthy additions to your meal with just the right kind of supplement for your gut microbiome.

- Bananas

This superfood contains plenty of dietary fibre essential for gut health and also forming easy to pass poop. Bananas also contain what is called fructo-oligosaccharide (FOS) which is a prebiotic. FOS is not broken down in the small intestines and makes its way to your large intestines where it is fermented in the colon thus adding to your good gut bacteria.

- Green leafy vegetables

Leafy greens and dark green vegetables are essentially one of the best for gut health as they are both rich in dietary fibre and vitamins and minerals. Eat plenty of greens to ensure you supplement your body with plenty of vitamin C, K, potassium, folate, and magnesium. Greens also provide your body with polyphenols which work as antioxidants essential for reducing inflammation, aiding cell renewal, and managing oxidative stress (which happens when free radicals which are unstable molecules in your body) increase and can lead to diseases such as cancer.

- Nuts

Almonds are known to benefit your gut bacteria and are just one of the types of nuts that benefit your body and your gut microbiome. Nuts too are rich sources of polyphenols and prebiotics helping your good bugs thrive.

- Berries

Berries contain polyphenols, vitamin C and lots of fibre. They are also rich in compounds that help stabilise the digestion process and the health of good gut bacteria. Raspberries and blackberries can provide you with close to 20% of your fibre requirements to ensure good bowel movements while vitamin C helps your gut with the absorption of iron.

Whether you are vegan, vegetarian, or love your meats, incorporating plenty of plant foods into your diet is not difficult. There are plenty of recipes out there catering to individual tastes.

Make Planning Easier With a Variety Checklist Magnet

Magnetic checklists are very handy tools to have on your fridge or any handy surface you can attach them to. Of course, having them on your fridge makes it easier to jot down ingredients you've run out of or just finished.

Next, let's look at more comprehensive methods to take care of your gut health. Simple and easy lifestyle changes that do not ask for extravagant expenditures.

Chapter 4:

Nourish Your Body

Time to start making your gut smile!

You will be surprised to learn that making your gut happy is one of the easiest and cheapest tasks you ever take on because no drastic and dramatic changes are required. Instead, I want to show you how a few simple and free lifestyle switches including changing up the way you eat, drink, play, and look at life in general are going to make a remarkable impact on your gut and overall health.

Let's look at initiating gradual and small changes, thus, avoiding sudden changes that cause stress to your system; learn to let go of negativities and embrace a positive outlook toward life. Follow these simple rules and learn to change a few simple factors that promise you a happy gut, happy microbiome, and a glowing healthy you!

Factors You Can Change Easily for a Happy Gut

- Regulate your food by paying attention to what you eat when you eat, and how you eat.
- Improve on and focus on a regular exercise regime or any form of proper physical activity.
- Learn to relax and take care of your physical and mental needs, and 'yes' that means making time for the loo,

instead of holding in your urge to pee or poop because you are just too busy.

- Get enough sleep; a vital component for maintaining gut health by giving your physical and mental self, time to heal, repair, and rest.

- Control your antibiotic intake, making sure to be mindful of damaging the delicate balance of your gut flora.

Start Fresh—Change the Way You Eat

Now, it's time for you to formulate a plan and start eating clean, incorporating all the good food value rules you have learned so far with all you are going to learn to ensure you optimise your well-being.

A healthy balance of all the essential macro and micro nutrients are needed to ensure your health, vitality and energy. But there are times we need to eat to simply feel good too by treating your dopamine induced reward system, to do so and still maintain a healthy eating habit you can follow the 80–20 split.

The 80% and 20% Eating Rule

- Eighty percent of the food you eat must be nutrient-dense. A good balance of carbs, proteins, fats, minerals, and vitamins to safeguard your gut flora and to overall health.

- Twenty percent of the food you eat can be calorie-dense. This number can be reduced but never exceeded. These are indulgent foods that have no nutritional benefit to your body and in some circumstances can cause harm. Therefore, such foods can be eaten or not as it does not make a favourable impact on your gut microbiome or overall health. High-sugar treats, alcohol and other types that are generally best left out or eaten in very limited quantities fall into this category.

Sticking to food that will benefit your gut bacteria to help increase the diversity of your gut flora is the wisest choice you can make and forgo the 80–20 rule. To do so, you need to make that connection with your gut, use the elimination test, and others to learn more about what makes up your microbiome in order to choose food that suits your unique gut bacteria.

Eat in Line With Your Biochemical Makeup

Keeping in line with your biochemical make-up which is made up of chemical compounds that put together your cells and other elements that decide on how your body functions, will help you to choose beneficial food types and avoid those that cause harm. To do so you must consider genetics, age, health standards, and gender, together with your lifestyle choices.

Since our genes are a 50:50 split of what we inherit from our mother and father, we cannot base our signature needs on our parents' biochemical make-up. Plus, we also learned that the gut microbiome is exceedingly diverse from person to person. Therefore, you need to look at your personal characteristics listed below.

Basing Your Food Choices on Genetics

Eating food that's compatible with your genes is gaining interest as research is helping scientists discover specific benefits in doing so as research has revealed improvements in gluten intolerance, weight loss, and insulin resistance (Xu et al.,

2013). To determine your genetic make-up, a simple DNA test is required. DNA alone is not substantial enough though for determining your unique food choices.

Food Choices Based on Gender

Hormones determine nutritional values between men and women. Oestrogen and progesterone of which females have a higher percentage change in levels depending on their menstruation cycles. The hormones also make females more sensitive toward calorie-reduced diets, predominantly cutting back on carbs.

Testosterone is the male dominant hormone and will not fluctuate but remains the same at all times. Due to this, men can tolerate various diets such as reduced-protein diets, low-carb eating plans and intermittent fasting.

Age and Diets

Age changes your body's requirements. For example, an older person will require less calories per day, but their nutritional needs will increase compared to their younger counterparts. A lower metabolism, and reduced activity are some of the factors while the diversity of the gut microbiome has been seen to reduce in people past the age of 60–65. Therefore, it's important to supplement probiotics and prebiotics and eat more gut friendly easy to digest food types.

It is more practical to focus on your biological age based on your mental and physical condition rather than your chronological age (number of years you have been alive) when determining your nutritional needs; most people feel different to their biological age in comparison to their chronological age.

One of the secrets to longevity and a healthy ageing pattern is to take care of your gut microbiota. Probiotics containing the lactic acid bacteria are found to be beneficial toward maintaining brain health, and the degeneration of one's cognitive functions is a symptom associated with ageing (Tooley, 2020). Therefore, taking care of your gut bacterial needs at any age will certainly have long-term benefits.

There was another study that confirmed ageing was more influenced by inflammation which became more pronounced as the quality of the gut microbiota starts to reduce (Wu et al., 2021). And went on to further clarify that the health of the gut microbiota in ageing people relied heavily on how rich and diverse their diets were.

Increasing your protein intake as you age is beneficial in retaining muscle mass, which you tend to lose at a faster rate when ageing. In addition, you will have to be more alert to food sensitivities and digestive problems that start to crop up as a result of your changing gut microbiome.

The best plan of action though is to start taking care of your gut microbiome and overall health with healthy, clean eating patterns which I will discuss more in this chapter.

Diet Based on Lifestyle

Your level of activity will determine the type of carbs, proteins and fats you require. If you are generally active, you will need a good balance of proteins and carbs, while an athlete who burns extra fuel will need extra carbs for energy and proteins to rebuild wasted muscles. The macronutrients your body requires must be determined by your lifestyle.

Balancing Blood Sugar Levels Through Sensible Eating

Eating carbs and sugars causes your digestive system to turn them into blood glucose. After which, your pancreas releases the hormone insulin, depending on the level of blood sugar in your system. Insulin helps your muscles, cells, and organs to digest the blood glucose and save it as fuel to be used when energy is needed.

While blood sugar is essentially fuel for your body, too much of a good thing can turn bad when you eat the wrong type of foods.

Carbs are the main contributors toward blood sugar, and the weaker the carb the faster your gut breaks it down, turning into sugar to be absorbed by your bloodstream as glucose. Just like a car, your body only requires a specific amount of fuel depending on how much you use.

If you lead a sedentary lifestyle and load up on carbs your blood sugar levels are going to go beyond the required amount. Therefore, once insulin is done storing glucose energy in your muscles and cells, it will go ahead and store the rest as fat to be used for a rainy day. That excess fat will only get used if you don't refresh your body with more carbs to turn into blood glucose. Sadly, we don't stop eating, unless of course we decide to fast.

Fasting for over 16-hours will deplete blood sugar levels in your cells and muscles and you will start to feel an energy slump, that's when your body starts to use the reserved energy stored as fat.

Sadly, most people keep eating and adding to their blood sugar and when insulin can't work fast enough to break down all the blood glucose the levels increase; having increased blood sugar levels long term puts you at risk of developing disease such as type-2 diabetes. You can of course manage falling into this troublesome cycle by avoiding the wrong type of carbs. Let's not forget the damage that elevated levels of blood sugar does to your gut bacteria; it leads to dysbiosis which is a marker for leaky gut.

Your Food Journal Can Help You Monitor Your Diet

If you are now concerned about what you are eating against what you should be eating, it's time to turn to your trusty old food journal for some added support. Here's what you can do.

- While jotting down your daily meals and food types for each meal you eat, go ahead and make a note of the macronutrients in the ingredients. That way, you can get an idea of the percentage of carbs, proteins, and fats you eat for a day.

    You can make tracking your macros a breeze by simply downloading an app that does it for you. MyFitnessPal and several others are out there for you to choose from.

- Observe how you feel after the meal. Have a little column on the side to jot down how the aftermath of the meal was; energised and then a crash, feeling sluggish, vitalized for longer, feeling hungry as though you didn't eat enough, or feeling full and satisfied until your next meal.

- It's important to make a note of the time you had the meal and for how long each meal kept you feeling full and satisfied and how long since eating before you started to feel hungry again. You will be able to observe a pattern related to certain food varieties. For example, carbs that are high in dietary fibres (whole grains, oats) will make you feel fuller for longer, while white bread or sugary doughnuts will make you feel hungry within a short time of eating them.

The main analysis you are looking for here are macro combinations that keep you feeling vitalized and full for longer, but there too, the quality of the macro will matter a lot because not all carbs, fats and proteins are a part of 'clean' ingredients.

Clean Eating and Maintaining the 80% to 20% Eating Rule

Eating with the pure intention of nourishing and energising your body is what clean eating is all about. It is not about eating bland or tasteless food or cutting calories. People who maintain a clean and wholesome way of eating enjoy delicious, filling, and nourishing meals minus the guilt and negative effects that follow eating too many calorie-dense meals.

When you choose to eat balanced meals you are choosing to eat from all food values carbs, proteins, fats, vitamins, and minerals.

Carbohydrates

These are essential for energy and are made up of the following:

- Dietary fibres—cannot be broken down by your small intestines and will travel to your large intestine to help bulk up your poop, making them into those healthy slightly firm sausage shapes you can easily pass.

    Fibres keep you feeling fuller for longer and aid your gut microbiome. Whole grains where the bran has not

116

been removed, brown rice, wheat, whole wheat pasta, fruits, vegetables are all healthy sources of dietary fibre. Fibre is also a source of food for your gut bacteria and will help increase the number of good bacteria in as little as two weeks of eating a diet rich in fibre. Soluble fibre mixes with water and helps to make your stool bulky and easy to pass. It also helps carry out LDL (bad) cholesterol from your body. Insoluble fibre turns to a gelatinous substance in your gut and helps food to pass along the intestines easily; it gets digested by the bacteria in your large intestines

- Sugars—natural sugars found in fruits and vegetables as fructose, dairy as lactose, and pure glucose found in honey, dried fruits, and fruit juices.

- Starch—end up getting converted into glucose by your digestive system. Grains, rice, potato, and sweet potato are sources of starch that get converted to glucose.

Carbohydrates You Must Avoid—Calorie Dense Food

Avoid all simple carbs; processed carbs including refined grains and sugars.

- Refined grains: White rice and grains where the bran is removed and the grains are polished; white flour and its by-products have very low fibre content and will get digested and converted to blood sugar very fast. The result; elevated blood glucose levels and feeling hungry sooner leading to over-eating. These foods are triggers for diabetes and obesity.

- Added sugars that have been extracted from their natural source thus changing their molecular structure are what's added to food to increase their sweetness.

They include table sugar, cane sugar, glucose, dextrose, sucrose; any added sugars that ends with 'ose' should be avoided and will be found in soft drinks, cakes, sweets, white bread, pastry, etc. (read the food value labels to find the percentage of added sugars in the food you buy). Honey and molasses are naturally occurring sugars but are classified as added sugars when they are added to enhance the sweetness of a meal. They are however more tolerated as healthier options.

Eating too many added sugars is bad.

- Raises triglyceride levels, (fat deposits in the blood and tissue) leading to heart disease.

- Increase blood sugar levels causing diabetes, obesity, and weight gain.

- Tooth decay caused by an increase of bad bacteria feeding on their favourite food—sugars.

Added sugars should not exceed 10% of your daily calories. A 2,000-calorie diet must have no more than 200 calories of added sugars. If you are considering heart health, bring the number down to just 100 calories of added sugar for a 2,000 calorie diet.

Did you know?

- One teaspoon of sugar equals 16 calories; 4 grams.

- 100 calories is 24 grams; therefore, no more than 6 teaspoons of sugar a day.

- 200 calories is 48 grams; therefore, no more than 12 teaspoons of sugar a day.

Shocking as it is, we often overeat sugars not knowing how much we are packing on with each teaspoon.

Proteins

Proteins are your body's building blocks and provide your body with essential amino acids needed for helping cells and muscles grow and repair.

- Lean meats
- Chicken
- Eggs
- Dairy
- Fruits
- Grains
- Seeds
- Nuts
- Tofu
- Seitan (wheat gluten popular among vegetarians as a rich source of protein)

You can load up on your daily protein requirements even if you are a vegan or vegetarian by eating plenty of protein-rich plant foods.

Proteins You Must Avoid

Processed meats are number one on the list. Avoid these as they are only calorie-dense and offer no nutritional value to your food. Sausages, bacon, and canned processed meats are a few of the examples.

Lots of red meat. Apart from choosing lean meats, try to avoid too many red meats; pork, beef, and lamb are examples. There are toxic compounds in red meat that are capable of harming your gut bacteria and causing changes in your microbiome. There are even links to red meat and cancer in the colon, obesity, kidney damage, diabetes and heart ailments.

Fats

Eat plenty of healthy fats. They include avocado, coconut, walnut, and olive oils. Stay away from the mass-produced industrial seed oils as they have the potential to turn carcinogenic at high heat. Butter and ghee are sources of animal fat you can enjoy in moderation as healthy lipids.

Minerals and Vitamins

Load up on plenty of fruits and vegetables to obtain essential vitamins and minerals. Remember the *5 colour fruit and veg a day* rule, and incorporate the habit into your new clean-eating regime.

Your gut flora produces essential vitamins and also thrives on vitamins and minerals obtained through the food you eat. These food values are essential to help the function of your immune system while maintaining the diversity of your gut flora.

Bottom line: Clean eating is about eating real food, food that has not been processed so much that their entire molecular structure is changed. I am talking about whole foods—fresh, bursting with nutrition and unprocessed.

Foods that have been mass produced and have been altered to look nothing like its original structure, like margarine which is vegetable seed oil that has been chemically changed to stay solid at room temperature and look like butter (when it's not), are fine examples of high-fat foods that should be avoided.

Food laden with too many additives and even fruit juices are not the ideal nutrients for you. Fruits that are juiced are devoid of their fibre and do not offer the same nutritional value as whole fruits. High-fat and high-sugar foods are capable of altering your gut microbiome and causing conditions like dysbiosis, leaky gut and inflammation.

The Benefits of Eating Whole Foods

Whole foods are what you include in your diet when you practice clean eating. They are packed with all the essential nutrients your body needs and managing them in the right quantities will not only support your gut microbiome but a number of other conditions.

Manage and Regulate Inflammation

Some of the best whole foods are plant-based varieties packed with lots of phytonutrients. We already covered the amazing effects of phytonutrients in Chapter 2, to which you can now add anti-inflammatory properties.

While you can manage inflammation purely on a vegetarian diet there are other sources of whole foods too that offer anti-inflammatory properties. The Mediterranean diet is a fine example where you can include the following foods that offer anti-inflammatory properties.

- Fatty fish
- Dark green leafy vegetables
- Nuts and seeds

- Fruits (colourful varieties like strawberries, oranges, blueberries, cherries)
- Turmeric
- Healthy fats
- Tomato

Common Inflammatory Foods to Avoid

- Refined carbs
- Industrial seed oils, that deliver more than the required value of omega-6 fatty acids
- Trans fats found in margarine, shortening and other hydrogenated oils
- Red meat including refined meats

Since we all possess unique biological structures, the types of foods that cause inflammation will differ from person to person. Therefore it's important to practise healthy habits to minimise inflammation triggers.

- Supplementing on omega-3 essential fatty acids to maintain a balance between omega-6s (linoleic acid). Omega-3 fatty acids are essential for brain and eye health and must be obtained through food or supplements offering essential eicosapentaenoic acid (EPA), and docosahexaenoic acid (DHA). Some foods like vegetable seed oils are high in omega-6 which is essential for heart health and reducing cholesterol but deadly in large doses as it triggers inflammation. The ideal ratio of omega-6 to omega 3 is 4:1; add 4 grams of omega 6 for every 1 gram of omega-3. Sadly, the typical western diet high in saturated fats often puts this ratio out of whack; consciously eating healthy fats and avoiding fast food is a good start to getting the balance in order.

- Drink adequate liquids to avoid dehydration.

- Maintain a healthy sleep schedule of at least seven to eight hours a night.

- Indulge in light exercise. Yoga, Tai Chi, brisk walks, swimming, an easy bike ride.

- Control your blood sugar levels.

Avoid Gluten

Gluten, a plant-based protein found in carbs can cause quite a bit of trouble and is found in most treats we love to eat such as white bread, pizza and cereals. You already know gluten is a high-risk factor for people with celiac disease. If you are dealing with chronic inflammation, it may make sense to switch to a gluten-free diet, avoiding markers that lead to not only inflammation but other syndromes triggered by the substance.

Take the 7-Day Gluten-Free Diet Test

Eliminate the least nutritious carbohydrates from your diet and try to be as gluten-free as possible for seven days and see how you feel.

- Avoid refined carbs
- Added sugars

- Modified fats
- White bread

Replace with.

- Leafy greens
- Sourdough bread
- Soaked whole grains
- Starchy vegetables (potato, beetroot, parsnip, pumpkin, carrots, kumara)

Avoid Excess Sugar

Sugars as discussed under carbohydrates when added to food become calorie-dense with no real nutritional value.

Why You Crave Sugars

You crave sugar mostly when you have trained your mind through short and long-term memory to associate the taste with your reward fulfilment system. Sugar also increases the secretion of serotonin, the neurotransmitter influencing your mood, appetite, memory, and levels of happiness; thus, associating eating sugar with feeling good. Your reward-seeking behaviour influences such cravings by telling you snacks at tea time are necessary, makes you crave a sweet after meals, and snacks while watching television, reading or relaxing.

While changing the way your mind reacts and craves sugar is possible through willful habits, the food you eat too can influence your sugar cravings. Insufficient protein and fat consumption are triggers.

Both macros slow down the absorption of sugars keeping cravings at bay for longer. It is similar to what happens when you eat simple carbs and it's metabolised too fast causing cravings and hunger too soon.

Low levels of blood sugar are another cause of sugar cravings. This happens often when you first cut out the simple carbs you have been eating. But in time, your body adjusts and starts to burn stored fats, thus regulating your energy levels.

Less sleep is another factor, as brain fatigue leaves you craving a quick energy boost, while stress and an increase of cortisol, the stress hormone, increases your hunger cravings.

Artificial Sweeteners Are Not All Good

These are much sweeter than sugars and offer zero calories causing no blood sugar spikes. But, artificial sweeteners can influence insulin secretion in small doses due to what is called 'cephalic phase insulin release', and some like aspartame can alter your gut microbiome with negative results and even a rise in blood sugar (Suez et al., 2014). The safest practice therefore, is eating sugars in moderation.

The Sugar Influenced Disease—Candida

A yeast fungus that lives in your gut and mouth, candida is harmless and aids your digestive function when in normal numbers. However, your diet and lifestyle can cause an increase of the fungus. Eating too many high-sugar foods and artificial sweeteners feeds candida which is kept suppressed by other gut bacteria.However, when your microbiome balance shifts due to various factors and the fungus is fed its favourite diet, you are in trouble of developing digestive problems such as bloating, or gastrointestinal disease.

Factors that help candida thrive are the same that cause dysbiosis and a weak gut flora, plus supplementing on too many sweets (natural and artificial) seals the deal. The good news is, cutting down on sugars and making lifestyle changes quickly wipes out the candida colonisation putting your gut flora back in balance.

Avoid Excess Caffeine

Too much caffeine, found most in coffee is not acceptable if you choose a wholesome diet. I get it, your daily mug of coffee is probably the motivation you need to get started and I am not going to put a damper on that!

Research regarding the pros and cons of coffee is still not conclusive, therefore for now practising moderation will be in your best health.

Why Too Much Coffee/Caffeine is Bad

Consuming over 400 g of caffeine a day can be bad.

- Effects of caffeine on your brain—Despite stimulating your central nervous system, too much caffeine can have the opposite effect and cause insomnia and fatigue.

- Headaches, dizziness, irritability caused by caffeine dependence and addiction due to caffeine's ability to increase your dopamine secretion; a neurotransmitter that influences the reward system.

- Dehydration occurs from coffee because caffeine is a diuretic; a substance that makes you lose water from your body. Therefore, you must replace one cup of coffee with two cups of water.

- Caffeine can increase blood pressure if you consume over four cups of coffee a day; a marker for cardiovascular disease.

- Caffeine triggers your pituitary gland to secrete adrenaline; a hormone associated with heightened levels of blood pressure.

- Caffeine impacts insulin levels and causes disruption with potential side effects of increased blood sugar levels.

- Caffeine causes gut problems as it stimulates stomach muscles to contract, causing pain, diarrhea, and increases the number of times you poop.

What's the Solution?

Get your energy fix from a different source!

Avoid all the negative baggage that comes with coffee (okay, you can still enjoy your morning mug!) and take a look at these alternative energy sources. Remember that the quick rush of energy coffee gives is temporary but the side effects will build and last longer.

- Supplements of quality multivitamins, minerals, wild fish oil, flaxseed oil, and coenzyme Q10 (CoQ10) to stimulate your hormone secretion, energise and make up for nutritional shortfalls.

Q10 is a co-enzyme present in all your cells; it aids with energy sustenance acting as an energy transport chain. Choose high -

quality fermented Q10 supplements for both stress management and energy boost.

Curb Your Alcohol Consumption

In Chapter 2, we discussed the role of alcohol in dysbiosis and liver disease; so, you already know it is not gut-friendly. Neither is it the best for maintaining a healthy diet.

Alcohol increases cortisol and insulin levels and causes blood sugar spikes. Alcohol can cause insulin resistance, putting you at risk of developing type-2 diabetes.

How to Avoid Excessive Alcohol Consumption?

- Associate relaxation with other methods. You can try yoga, mindful meditation, walks or spending time with friends who are not dependent on alcohol for a good time.

- Choose non-alcoholic beverages when you go out. If you must imbibe, alternate between the two so you don't overdo it.

- Avoid social pressure to drink. Know your needs and limits and stick to them.

- Avoid drinking other than for social occasions; limiting alcohol consumption to no more than two or four units.

- Choose red wine over hard liquor but in moderation. Red wine is high in antioxidants and other benefits but is certainly not a health supplement, merely a better alternative to most other liquor.

The Importance of Proper Hydration

Proper hydration is essential for a healthy body. Your body is over 60% water, while most of your organs contain a larger percentage of water (Water Science School, 2019).

- Brain and heart—73% water
- Lungs—83% water
- Muscle and kidney—83% water

To keep these organs functioning well, it's essential to drink enough liquids. Therefore, you need to make it a habit to drink water throughout the day and not when you are thirsty. The recommended requirements of water by gender are as follows.

Males—3.7 litres a day

Females—2.7 litres

Aiming to drink more is even better, while more active individuals and athletes should drink close to 5 litres a day. Water is not the only source of hydration; vegetables and fruits also contain fair amounts of liquids and offer around 20% of liquid intake a day.

How Do I Know I'm Dehydrated?—Look for the Signs

- Dark colored urine that smells.
- A dry feeling in the mouth and parched lips.
- Suffering from lethargy
- Needing to pass urine less than four times a day.

Must I Only Drink Water?

Not at all. As long as you load up on healthy liquids it does not have to be water, although there is nothing quite as exhilarating as a glass of cool water when you are thirsty. Try these water substitutes.

- Green tea
- Vegetable juice
- Berry-infused water—slice up your favourite berries and add them to a jug of water and drink throughout the day.
- Lemon water
- Milk
- Sparkling water

Best Type of Water to Drink

Do avoid drinking from plastic bottles. A chemical known as phthalates present in plastic can often seep through the plastic and get into the water you drink. The probability is higher when the bottle gets heated.

- Spring water contains natural minerals.
- Distilled water (ionised water).
- Tap water where the pH level is constantly monitored.

Now, let's fine-tune the process more by incorporating a few healthy habits that will complete your overall transformation to a healthier, happier body, mind, and soul.

Chapter 5:

Honour Your Body and Mind

Daily habits that make your life stress free are the foundation to leading a healthy life. When you are happy and confident in life, it gives you the strength to initiate change and take on challenges.

Let's look at subtle changes you can make to the way you conduct your daily routines, tasks, and chores; changing aspects that are within your control is the first step toward a healthier outlook in life.

Practice Mindful Eating

Mindful eating quite simply is to prepare and eat your meals consciously.

Paying attention to the act of eating and making it an almost spiritual experience will make the food you prepare, or buy, and eat all the more special. Best of all, it's an immersive and fun experience you are going to be looking forward to as the time you spend preparing and eating your meal is solely focused on nurturing your body and treating your tastebuds; it's a wonderful method of decompressing and turning your thoughts away from daily stresses.

What Are the Benefits?

- Becoming conscious of your food choices, thus making you question reaching out for unhealthy food choices.

- Learning to slow down; no multitasking in between meals.

- Enjoy the experience and learn to appreciate and savour the flavours, aroma, and sensation of everything you eat.

- You learn to celebrate the meal you are eating and feel pleasure in doing so.

- You are more relaxed thus aiding the digestion process, you are not eating while stressing over work, and other things that can cause hormone fluctuations, instead you are centred on the eating experience and your gut-brain axis is working together focused solely on the digestion process.

- Avoid overeating because you are conscious of your stomach filling up and you feel fuller sooner and more satisfied.

How to Practise Mindful Eating

1. Start small, with the preparation of a snack. Once you get the hang of it, you may progress to other meals. Plan to prepare your meals at home more than eating out. Think about the ingredients and their benefits based on what you have learned. Increase the time you spend in the kitchen associating the space as a spot for decompressing and treating yourself to nourishment.

2. Go slow, once your meal is set up in front of you don't start eating immediately. Pay attention to how it looks, the colours, and the aroma.

3. Pop the first bite in your mouth and try to identify the flavours, let the taste of spices and herbs you added come through. Savour the texture of the food on your tongue as you chew slowly.

4. Notice how you start to feel, if you are hungry be conscious of how that hunger is getting filled, how with every bite you are starting to feel fuller. Be very aware of chewing your food and rolling it around on your tongue to savour the flavours before swallowing, don't let it be an automatic response.

Practice mindful eating at every meal and you will soon begin to feel the difference both physically and mentally; creating a deeper connection between your mind and your body to feel complete and happy after each meal.

Pay Attention to How Much You Move

Physical activity is essential to optimise the gut-brain axis; your brain requires the most energy to function together with other organs. The mitochondria which is responsible for the generation of cells to aid your mental and physical functions need an endless supply of energy to function flawlessly.

Food that is digested is your body's primary and essential source of energy. Supplements compensate only a minute percentage. Both food and supplements must first be digested and absorbed to offer your body the nutrients they contain and your digestive tract is the only system to aid this function.

Bottom line: you need a well-functioning digestive tract to feel physically fit and to indulge in physical exercise. If you lack the energy, you cannot perform any form of energy-expending actions. Therefore, nurturing your gut to optimise the absorption of nutrients is what is going to keep your energy levels up.

Times Your Gut Health is Causing Your Energy Slump

The usual digestive problems we face are often the culprits. You know what they are by now; indigestion, bloating, gas.

Look for the signs.

- Bad breath, craving sweets, mood alterations, skin allergies, and any other significant changes.

Other reasons for an energy slump and poor digestion include.

- Inflammation
- Zinc deficiency
- The ageing process

Avoid energy slumps by optimising food absorption and your digestive process by supplementing and adding food containing the following vitamins and minerals.

- Vitamin B-1, B-2, B-5, and B-12
- Magnesium
- Zinc
- Supplement of probiotics

- Supplement of digestive enzymes
- Paying attention to the preparation of more gut-friendly food types is an added boost.

Exercise and Enjoy Movement

Celebrate being active. Even if you do not like the concept of exercise, you can ditch the gym sessions and look for other forms of physical activity to keep your body moving. There are plenty of options out there to optimise your gut health; crunches, dancing classes, yoga, swimming, biking, weekend treks with friends, tai chi in the park; be creative, and look for activities you love.

How to Get Motivated to Get Moving

- Find your reason to get moving—health, socialising, getting rid of boredom; the reasons are endless.
- Find a friend to partner up with
- Embrace physical activity and don't be embarrassed
- Enjoy being flexible
- Make exercise a daily routine
- Listen to the needs of your body
- Try new things
- Practise mindful breathing

Yoga Movements to Improve Your Gut

Yoga is not an activity to feel intimidated by. Those super flexible poses you see people practice come from years of following the exercise. No elaborate moves are expected from beginners in a yoga class. So, do make the effort, if you are even slightly interested, to sign up for a gut-healthy yoga class.

Yoga Poses That Help Digestion

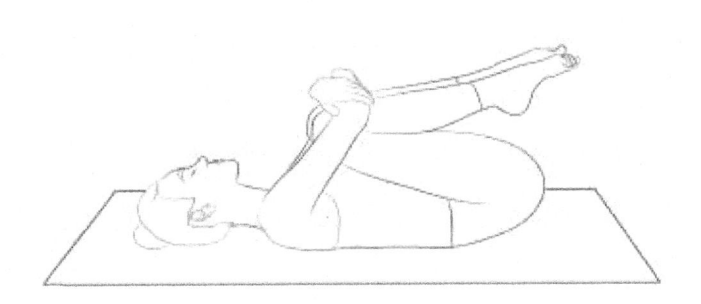

- Knees to chest *apanasana*

knees to chest apanasana

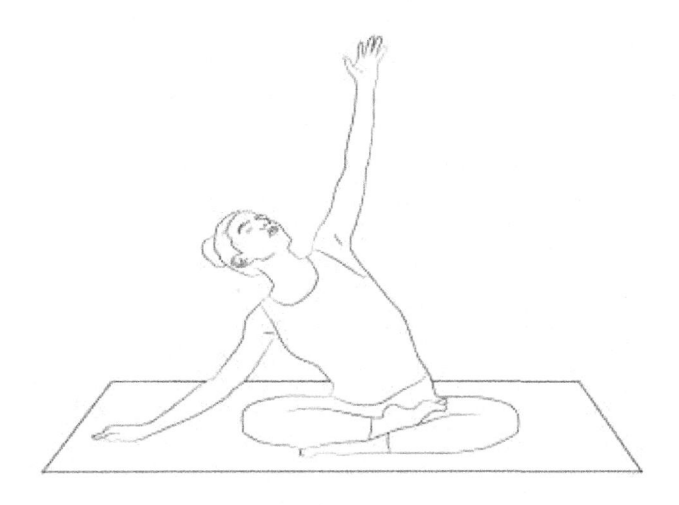

- Seated side bend *parsva sukhasana*

- Cat-cow pose *marjaryasana-bitilasana*

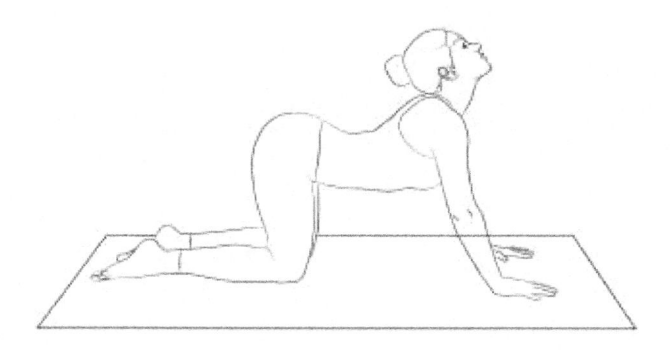

cat pose marjaryasana-bitilasana

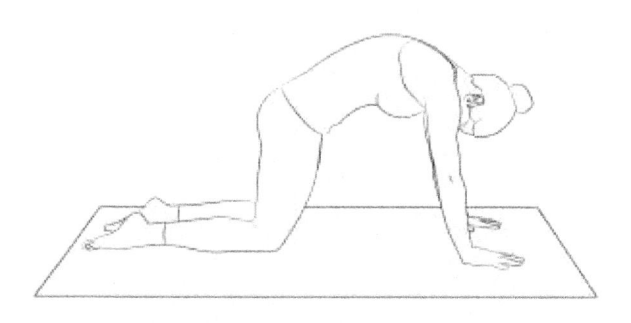

cow pose marjaryasana-bitilasana

- Bow pose *dhanurasana*

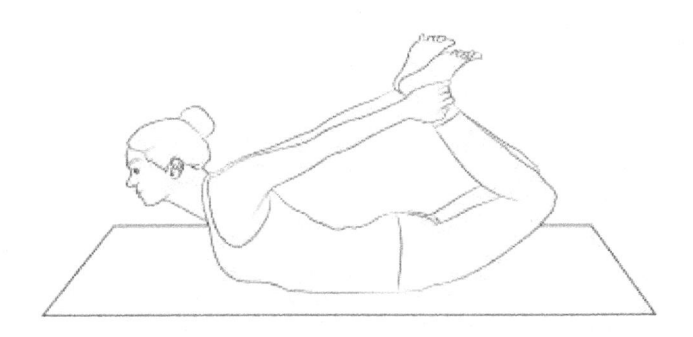

bow pose dhanurasana

- Seated twist *ardha matsyendrasana*

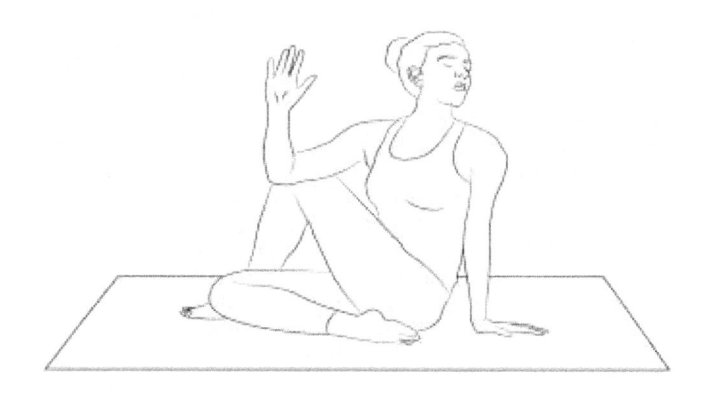

seated twist ardha matsyendrasana

Practising yoga at home in front of a mirror is one way to get started. You will find plenty of tutorial videos online that you can follow to master each pose.

Deep Breathing Guide

Mindful breathing is when you practise deep breathing from your abdomen, just like a newborn baby does. If you watch one, you will see their stomachs rise and fall, instead of their chest. Even adults breathe this way when they are asleep and at rest.

Consciously breathing to expand your belly and fill your lungs with air is soothing and relaxing. Best of all, you can practice deep breathing anywhere; at the office, before bedtime, or on a park bench. Any place you feel comfortable practising deep breathing is ideal, simply follow the given steps.

- Sit comfortably, or lie down

- Place a hand on your chest and on your abdomen

- Inhale deeply through your nose, and let your stomach bloat so your hand moves up. Your chest must move only slightly or not at all.

- Exhale from your mouth, and watch your stomach fall back down.

- Practise inhaling and exhaling until you get the hang of it.

- Now, breathe in and count, starting with one. As you exhale, say 'calm' and focus on the keyword; block out any other thoughts.

- Repeat ten times and feel a warm sense of peace take over.

Yoga and breathing are beneficial for soothing and improving the function of your digestive system. A combination of both techniques may even have long-term benefits, helping to keep conditions like leaky gut at bay.

It's time for change, a big step, but one that I am confident you are ready to make. And since your entire wellness is centred around your digestive tract, it's time to initiate that change in the first place that influences your gut—your kitchen.

Chapter 6:
Create Your Wholesome Kitchen

You may not realise it but most of your eating practices are centred on habits. Norms you cultivated from childhood as they were instilled in you by your parents as good and necessary routines.

Habits are familiar and strangely comforting which is why most people are reluctant to change, even when they are presented with healthier alternatives. Plus, our minds are hardwired into thinking we 'need' certain foods, ingredients and quantities to make our meals a success. For example, the habit of eating breakfast, lunch, and dinner is a modern myth cultivated by a generation that suddenly had a surplus of food and didn't know what to do with it. Think back, your hunter-gatherer ancestors ate when food was available and fasted when there was none; they survived and thrived to bring us into this modern age, minus the chronic diseases too, which seems to be another affliction of modern society.

Change is challenging but it can be achieved by taking easy baby steps toward your goals. First, make that resolve to choose health and happiness. Start making simple shifts in the way you prepare meals and the way you eat; start by trying new and easy recipes.

Think about all the nutritious options you can include in your diet and all the harmful elements you can take out. Do not dwell on the past and the harmful food you ate, this is your chance for a fresh start.

How to Get Started—Creating Your Wholesome Kitchen

Planning ahead is crucial to avoid last minute triggers that make you choose unhealthy eating options simply because it is the easier option. Therefore, start with a stock of healthy essentials; ingredients that help you to throw a meal together without having to resort to the pre-cooked, processed versions.

Look at stocking up on whole foods; canned vegetables can be easily replaced with washed and pre-cut fresh vegetables you can store in the freezer. A boiled chicken breast, when frozen, can be defrosted, flaked and used for bakes. Pasta or sandwiches instead of sausages or luncheon meat. When you stock up, concentrate on clean eating options that are nutrient dense and energising.

Putting Together a Nutrient-Dense Kitchen—What are the Staples?

Let's look at creating a wholesome pantry of essential food types that will support your gut and overall fitness—a detox from all the bad food you have been eating.

May I suggest you first take stock of your pantry and get rid of all unhealthy food stuff. The less there is, the less temptation. Having a big bowl of fruits in your kitchen is a good way to encourage yourself and the rest of the family to eat healthy snacks. Fruits and nuts and jugs of fruit or berry-infused cool water in the refrigerator can easily replace crisps, and soft drinks as go-to food whenever anyone gets the munchies.

Healthy Fats

Healthy fats can be divided by their smoke point, which is how long they take to heat up and start burning, which is when you see smoke rising from the oil.

Fats that have a higher smoke point are better for cooking as they do not heat up fast which causes certain chemical changes to take place in the oil including oxidation and alterations in the fatty acid compounds.

Healthy fats suited for cooking

- Extra virgin white coconut oil
- Lard
- Ghee which is clarified butter
- Avocado oil
- Tallow
- Grass fed organic butter can be used for cooking on a medium heat
- Olive oil has a low smoke point and is better for quick sautés and as a garnish.

Healthy Grains

The following whole grains, while being high in fibre and absolutely gut-friendly, are also gluten-free options that you can have in your pantry for putting a meal together.

Quinoa—this grain, whether you prefer the white or red variety, is high in proteins and contains several key amino acids which help develop your cells and muscles. Quinoa is a popular anti-inflammatory food.

Brown rice—from which the bran has not been removed, is high in dietary fibre and will feed your gut bacteria as it ferments in your large intestines and will also keep you feeling fuller for longer, unlike the white rice varieties which are simple carbs and easily cause blood sugar spikes. Brown rice contains protein, magnesium, vitamin-B1 or thiamine and calcium.

Millet—this grain is a prebiotic that is a good fertiliser for your good gut bacteria. A particularly digestive-healthy food, millet contains small levels of serotonin which is helpful for regulating and calming one's mood and helping with a good night's sleep.

Rolled oats—oats are great for controlling your blood sugar levels and contain both soluble and insoluble fibre.

Buckwheat—is an antioxidant and an anti-inflammatory. Its qualities include being heart healthy, helps with managing diabetes and contains fibre, protein and increases energy levels.

Healthy Legumes

Chickpeas—rich in protein and fibre help with insulin sensitivity and thus controlling blood sugar levels. A versatile legume to have in your kitchen chickpeas can be used to make hummus, salads or even a savoury snack.

Lentils—one of the best plant-based proteins, lentils are rich in zinc, iron, and vitamin B1. Having a jar of lentils at home will help you to create hearty winter warmer meals in double quick time. Just a quick lentil curry spooned over a bed of rice or eaten with brown bread is quite a wholesome and comforting meal.

Kidney Beans—these popular legumes are heart-healthy and may reduce blood pressure. Kidney beans contain proteins, carbs, and folate as well as thiamin among other essential minerals and vitamins.

Peas—antioxidant peas are high in protein and fibre. Helping to stabilise blood sugar levels, peas are a gut bacteria friendly food.

Soybeans—this is a very versatile bean that is high in protein and even believed to aid with reducing the risks of cancer although studies are still inconclusive.

Dairy and Alternatives

- Milk is gluten-free and rich in protein, fibre, and calcium. However, flavoured milk and cheeses which have been processed can contain gluten. Therefore, it's important to check the labels before you consume any type of dairy that has been processed.
- Coconut yoghurt
- Coconut milk

Healthy Nuts to Have as Snacks

- Chia seeds
- Pumpkin seeds
- Sesame seeds
- Almonds
- Raw cashew
- Raw Brazil nuts

- Raw walnuts

Nut Butters

Choose organic and whole-nut butters that do not contain added sugars.

- Almond butter
- Natural peanut butter

What's the Deal With Organic Produce?

Crops that are cultivated minus chemical fertilisers, synthetic growing agents, and irradiation, a type of radiation that helps to kill bacteria in crops, and are free from the influences of biotechnology are classified as organic.

Animals raised on organic feed and not kept in pens or coops, such as free-range chickens, pasture-fed and grass-fed cattle all fall into a similar 'organic' category. All this extra effort put into growing and raising organic produce makes them healthier and cleaner options but more expensive.

That's why the dirty and clean list has been created to help you know and choose between food that can be easily contaminated by chemicals and those that have thicker skins or are better protected from harmful toxins and are safer to eat.

I recommend you choose as much organic foods as you can afford and non-organics from the 'clean list'. One rule though is to thoroughly wash your fruit and veg before consumption, no matter which category they belong to.

Most Contaminated Produce—The Dirty Dozen

- Spinach
- Strawberries
- Kale, Mustard greens, and collards
- Celery
- Peaches
- Apples
- Capsicum, bell, hot peppers
- Cherries
- Pears
- Tomato
- Nectarines
- Grapes

The Least Contaminated—The Clean Fifteen

- Sweetcorn
- Pineapple
- Avocado
- Onions

- Papaya
- Frozen sweet peas
- Kiwi
- Honeydew melon
- Asparagus
- Cantaloupe Melon
- Mushroom
- Cabbage
- Sweet potato
- Watermelon
- Mangoes

Next, let's look at some quick recipes that will help you combine the best of these ingredients into delicious and wholesome meals.

Chapter 7:

Treat Your Tummy to Tasty Recipes

The recipes included in this chapter are oldies but goodies. Gut-healthy meals that are easy to whip up packed with nutrition and taste. Before we begin, here are some handy food hacks to keep in mind.

Healthy Food Hacks

- Pair turmeric with black pepper. Curcumin in turmeric is an anti-inflammatory compound but for your body to absorb it, curcumin must be combined with piperine found in black pepper, and a healthy fat.

- Diffuse harmful nitrates with some Vitamin C. Deli meats and other cured meats containing harmful nitrosamines can be diffused by combining them with antioxidants such as vitamin-C-containing food.

- Help proteins in meat digest faster with kiwi fruit; a natural enzyme kiwi when combined with meats such as steak helps you feel less full after the meal. Plus, it's a delicious combination.

- Drizzle lime or lemon juice over your greens to help the absorption of its iron better.

- Help fat soluble vitamins like A, K, E and D get better absorbed by eating veggies with a healthy fat.

- Preserve phytochemicals in veggies better by steaming them and not boiling.

Healthy Recipes

The following few recipes are just a sample for you to understand the scope of eating healthy. The variety and flavours are endless and nothing short of enjoyable.

Recipe No 1: Overnight Oats—Grab and Go Breakfast for Busy Mornings

Oats are gluten-free, heart-healthy and full of fibre. Overnight oats are even better as they remain uncooked and unchanged by heat and are super fast and easy to make.

Time: Total preparation time 8–10 hours

Serving Size: 1 portion

Prep Time: 15 minutes

Cook Time: none

Nutritional Facts/Info:

Calories	Carbs	Fat	Protein	Fibre
253	32 g	6 g	18 g	6 g

Ingredients:

- ⅓ cup gluten-free rolled oats
- ¾ cup any unsweetened plant-based milk like almond milk
- 2 Scoops vanilla-flavoured plant-protein powder
- 1 tbsp. walnuts crushed
- 1 tsp. chia seeds
- 1/4 tsp. cinnamon powder
- 1 small or ½ a medium banana sliced

Method:

Make the previous night. Add all ingredients in a glass bowl and give it a good stir. You can cover the bowl with cling film and place it in the refrigerator or spoon the mix into a mason jar, screw on the lid and chill. Simply pop the mason jar in your bag on your way out the next morning or enjoy it at leisure sitting by your sunny kitchen window.

Change up the ingredients as you go and enjoy variety.

Recipe No 2: Protein Fruit Smoothie

A quick energising breakfast you can make in seconds, protein shakes are a healthy start to your day, plus protein keeps you feeling fuller for longer.

Time: Total preparation time 10 minutes

Serving Size: 1 portion

Prep Time: 15 minutes

Cook Time: none

Nutritional Facts/Info:

Calories	Carbs	Fat	Protein	Fibre
60	16 g	13 g	24 g	4 g

Ingredients:

- 275 ml water or a plant-based milk (almond/rice/coconut)
- ½ Avocado, or 1 tbsp. healthy nut butter pecans, almond or coconut cream
- 25 g Fresh or frozen fruits. Choose those low on the glycemic index which means they will not cause immediate blood sugar spikes. Green apples, plums, cherries, dark berries, etc.

- 1 fistful of greens: Kale, spinach, and other dark green leafy varieties
- 2 scoops plant-based protein powder
- For sprinkling: coconut flakes, flax seeds, chia seeds

Method:

Add all ingredients in a blender and blitz until well combined. Sprinkle with the seeds/flakes and enjoy chilled.

Recipe No 3: Butternut Squash and Kale Soup

There is nothing quite like a warm and hearty soup packed with loads of nutritional goodness. This one is sure to be a family favourite that can be easily made with a bunch of leftover veg from your fridge.

Time: 45 minutes

Serving Size: 4–5 servings

Prep Time: 10 minutes

Cook Time: 35 minutes

Nutritional Facts/Info:

Calories	Carbs	Fat	Protein	Fibre
130	24 g	3.5 g	5 g	4 g

Ingredients:

- 2 tbsp. Extra virgin olive oil
- 2 Large butternut squash peeled and cubed enough to fill 6–8 cups in total
- 1 Medium onion diced
- 3 Cloves minced garlic
- 1 tbsp. Smoked paprika
- 1 tbsp. Cinnamon powder
- 4 cups vegetable broth (choose the gut healthy varieties)
- ¼ cup Unsweetened almond milk
- 2 tbsp. White coconut oil
- 1 Bunch kale

Method:

1. Get the oven going. Preheat to 200 degrees celsius.
2. Place diced squash on a baking tray and rub with the olive oil. Sprinkle it with salt and pop it in the oven for 40 minutes or until the squash is soft. Once done, set aside.
3. Place a large heavy bottomed soup pan on a medium heat and add coconut oil, once it's heated, add the onions and temper for about 5 minutes until soft and translucent. Next, add the garlic and stir fry for another 2–3 minutes.
4. Next, add the squash, cinnamon, paprika and the stock. Increase the heat a bit and bring it to a boil. Then reduce the heat and let it simmer for about 10–15 minutes. Enjoy the heavenly wafts of the soup as it fills your kitchen

5. Once done, add the almond milk and blend. You can use a stick blender and puree the soup until smooth, right in the pan. Or use a regular blender.
6. Add the kale and blend again. Season with salt and pepper to taste.
7. Serve warm with toasted whole wheat or sourdough bread. Enjoy.

Recipe No 4: Burrito Bowls With Chicken

Delightfully filling and packed with a range of flavours, this meal is going to be a big hit with the family and you. Feel proud serving this meal which has a combination of all the essential carbs, proteins, and fats. It's a full meal that is super easy to make too.

Time: 45 minutes

Serving Size: 4 servings

Prep Time: 10 minutes

Cook Time: 35 minutes

Nutritional Facts/Info:

Calories	Carbs	Fat	Protein	Fibre
685	64 g	25 g	45 g	10 g

Ingredients:

- ½ cup Uncooked quinoa
- ½ Can black beans
- 1 cup Organic vegetable broth
- 1 Medium red onion finely sliced
- ½ cup pineapple cut into small cubes
- 1 Medium-sized jalapeno pepper, deseeded, and chopped
- Juice of ½ a lime
- ⅛ cup Coriander leaves/cilantro
- 1 medium bell pepper cut into strips
- ½ tbsp. Extra virgin olive oil
- ¼ tsp. chilli powder
- ⅛ tsp. paprika powder
- ½ cup cooked and diced chicken breast
- ¼ cup plain Greek yoghurt
- 1 cup Baby spinach cut into strips
- 1 large Avocado sliced

Method:

1. Place a medium-size pan on a medium-low heat, add the vegetable stock and the quinoa and bring to boil then turn down the heat. Cover and let it simmer for about 12-15 minutes until the quinoa has soaked up all the broth.

2. Drain water from the beans, rinse them, and place in a bowl to warm up with some stock spooned over. You can microwave them for 1–2 minutes. Or in a pan on the stove.
3. While that's going, get yourself a small bowl and combine the pineapple, jalapeno, coriander (keep some for the garnish), half of the red onions, and lime juice.
4. Add the olive oil to a skillet that you warm up on medium heat and then add the remaining onions, peppers, chilli powder and paprika. Stir fry for about five minutes until the peppers become soft and your onions translucent.
5. Now you are ready to plate up. Into a serving bowl, spoon in a single portion of quinoa, then spoon over a portion of the beans, and the onions, peppers, and the cooked chicken and spinach. Spoon over the pineapple salsa and place a few slices of avocado on the side. Add a dollop of Greek yoghurt and some coriander leaves.
6. Enjoy your wholesome meal bursting with flavour!

Watch Out for More!

If you found these recipes useful and delicious options, watch out for more in my special anti-inflammatory diet cookbook coming soon.

Conclusion

As we come to the end of your journey through your amazing digestive tract, I hope you enjoyed the ride? The twists, the turns, and little stops along the way to meet your gut microbiome and learn more about the bacteria there. You are now more sensitive to your digestive tract and its needs; to what makes it tick, what makes it happy and what can cause it harm.

When your gut is happy, you are happy. That is a fact we have established through this journey learning about the most important system in your body.

And now it's time for the moment of truth, when you go out there and make that amazing change; not giant leaps but baby steps in the right direction.

Remember a healthy gut is a healthy you!

Stay in Touch

I would love to hear your thoughts about my book; I hope you enjoyed reading it as much as I did writing it for you. Please visit me at www.getyoursassyback.co.uk or on my Instagram account @getyoursassyback as well as my other social media platforms.

Let me know what you think about the information, how much you learned, and whether my book was eye-opening and motivated you to seek that all-important change you knew was needed but didn't know how to achieve. My friend, look after yourself. You are important.

Thank you!

References

3 Ways Our Gut Health Influences Our Weight. (n.d.). BePure Wellness. Retrieved July 19, 2022, from https://bepure.co.nz/blog/3-ways-our-gut-health-influences-our-weight/?_pos=47&_sid=3071c3e12&_ss=r

5 Fermented Foods for Great Gut Health. (n.d.). BePure Wellness. Retrieved July 23, 2022, from https://bepure.co.nz/5-great-foods-gut-health

7 Food Hacks to Get the Most Out of Your Food. (n.d.). BePure Wellness. Retrieved July 27, 2022, from https://bepure.co.nz/hacks-get-most-from-food

Andy. (2020). *What Is The Gut? Biology Lesson Time.* The Gut Stuff. https://thegutstuff.com/intro-to-the-gut/get-to-know-the-gut/

Anthenelli, R., & Grandison, L. (2012). Effects of stress on alcohol consumption. *Alcohol Research: Current Reviews, 34*(4), 381–382. https://www.ncbi.nlm.nih.gov/pmc/articles/PMC3860387/

Are You Eating Right For You? (n.d.). BePure Wellness. Retrieved July 22, 2022, from https://bepure.co.nz/eating-right-for-you

Azvolinsky, A. (2015, April). *Gut Microbes Influence Circadian Clock.* The Scientist Magazine®. https://www.the-scientist.com/daily-news/gut-microbes-influence-circadian-clock-35619

B, E. (2021, June 22). *The Signs of a Healthy Gut - KnowYourDNA*. Know Your DNA. https://knowyourdna.com/signs-of-healthy-gut/

BalistreriAugust 4, E., & read, 2020| 5 Mi. (2020, August). *The real reason it's so hard to quit eating sugar.* Www.tristarwell.com. https://www.tristarwell.com/insights/the-real-reason-its-so-hard-to-quit-eating-sugar

Berry, D. S., Spector, P. T., & Wolf, J. (2020, October). *The gut microbiome.* Joinzoe.com. https://joinzoe.com/whitepapers/gut-microbiome

Bjarnadottir, A. (2019, June 19). *Mindful Eating 101 — A Beginner's Guide.* Healthline. https://www.healthline.com/nutrition/mindful-eating-guide#rationale

Brazzier, Y. (2020, December 10). *Food Intolerance: Causes, types, symptoms, and diagnosis.* Www.medicalnewstoday.com. https://www.medicalnewstoday.com/articles/263965#symptoms

Britannica. (2019). Faeces | biology | Britannica. In *Encyclopædia Britannica.* https://www.britannica.com/science/feces

Campos-Rodríguez, R., Godínez-Victoria, M., Abarca-Rojano, E., Pacheco-Yépez, J., Reyna-Garfias, H., Barbosa-Cabrera, R. E., & Drago-Serrano, M. E. (2013). Stress modulates intestinal secretory immunoglobulin A. *Frontiers in Integrative Neuroscience*, *7*(86). https://doi.org/10.3389/fnint.2013.00086

CDC. (2019). *CDC -What is inflammatory bowel disease (IBD)? - Inflammatory Bowel Disease - Division of Population Health.* CDC. https://www.cdc.gov/ibd/what-is-ibd.htm

Churney, K. (2021, October 29). *Microbiome Testing Explained, Reviewed, & Questions Answered.* Healthline. https://www.healthline.com/health/microbiome-testing

Cleveland Clinic. (2021, August 12). *Colon (Large Intestine): Function, Anatomy & Definition.* Cleveland Clinic. https://my.clevelandclinic.org/health/body/22134-colon-large-intestine

CNN, S. L. (2022, April 7). *Dirty Dozen 2022: Produce with the most and least pesticides.* CNN. https://edition.cnn.com/2022/04/07/health/dirty-dozen-produce-2022-wellness/index.html

CSCS, M. M., MS. (2022, March 17). *Omega-6 to Omega-3 Ratio: What Does It Mean and What's Optimal?* Blog.insidetracker.com. https://blog.insidetracker.com/omega-6-omega-3-ratio

Dresden, D. (2022, April 18). *What to know about microbiome testing.* Www.medicalnewstoday.com. https://www.medicalnewstoday.com/articles/microbiome-testing#what-they-measure

Duyvestyn, H. (n.d.). *Nurturing Mindfulness Around Eating.* BePure Wellness. Retrieved July 23, 2022, from https://bepure.co.nz/mindful-eating

Edermaniger, L. (2019, October 17). *The Ultimate Guide To Polyphenols For Health And Gut Microbiome.* Atlas Biomed Blog | Take Control of Your Health with No-Nonsense News on Lifestyle, Gut Microbes and Genetics. https://atlasbiomed.com/blog/the-ultimate-guide-to-polyphenols-health-and-gut-microbiome/

Enterotype - an overview | ScienceDirect Topics. (2019). Www.sciencedirect.com.

https://www.sciencedirect.com/topics/immunology-and-microbiology/enterotype

ESNM. (2021, October 13). *Is healthy ageing and increased longevity connected to the gut microbiome?* Gut Microbiota for Health. https://www.gutmicrobiotaforhealth.com/is-healthy-aging-and-increased-longevity-connected-to-the-gut-microbiome/

Exploring the Perfect Diet for Your Genes. (2010, August 2). The Dr. Oz Show. https://www.drozshow.com/article/exploring-perfect-diet-your-genes

F. Moraes, A. C., de Almeida-Pittito, B., & Ferreira, S. R. G. (2019, January 1). *Chapter 41 - The Gut Microbiome in Vegetarians* (J. Faintuch & S. Faintuch, Eds.). ScienceDirect; Academic Press. https://www.sciencedirect.com/science/article/pii/B9780128152492000415

Gut health check: 5 signs of a healthy gut. (n.d.). Joinzoe.com. https://joinzoe.com/post/5-healthy-gut-signs

Gut microbes shape our antibodies before we are infected by pathogens. (2020, July 5). ScienceDaily. https://www.sciencedaily.com/releases/2020/08/200805124038.htm

Hansen, A. (n.d.). *Is a poop a day necessary for good health? Five experts have the same answer.* Quartz. https://qz.com/quartzy/1384812/how-often-should-you-poop-its-all-about-the-three-and-three-rule/

Harvard Health Publishing. (2017, April 12). *Ditch the Gluten, Improve Your Health? - Harvard Health.* Harvard Health; Harvard Health.

https://www.health.harvard.edu/staying-healthy/ditch-the-gluten-improve-your-health

Harvard Health Publishing. (2018, November 7). *Foods that fight inflammation - Harvard Health*. Harvard Health; Harvard Health. https://www.health.harvard.edu/staying-healthy/foods-that-fight-inflammation

Heiman, M. L., & Greenway, F. L. (2016). A healthy gastrointestinal microbiome is dependent on dietary diversity. *Molecular Metabolism*, 5(5), 317–320. https://doi.org/10.1016/j.molmet.2016.02.005

Hicklin, T. (2017, December 4). *Changing gut bacteria in Crohn's disease*. National Institutes of Health (NIH). https://www.nih.gov/news-events/nih-research-matters/changing-gut-bacteria-crohns-disease

How is Alcohol Really Affecting Your Health? (n.d.). BePure Wellness. Retrieved July 23, 2022, from https://bepure.co.nz/how-alcohol-really-affects-health?_pos=1&_sid=f523a9d68&_ss=r

How long is too long on the potty. (2017, November 1). Www.geisinger.org. https://www.geisinger.org/health-and-wellness/wellness-articles/2017/10/27/15/44/poop-or-get-off-the-potty

How To Create A Wholesome Kitchen. (n.d.). BePure Wellness. Retrieved July 26, 2022, from https://bepure.co.nz/bepure-handy-cupboard-items?_pos=6&_sid=b90cb8ee8&_ss=r

How to Diversify Your Diet. (n.d.). Pendulum. Retrieved July 13, 2022, from https://pendulumlife.com/blogs/news/how-to-diversify-your-diet

https://facebook.com/robinberzinmd. (2019, March 14). *mindbodygreen*. Mindbodygreen. https://www.mindbodygreen.com/0-12540/the-simple-elimination-diet-that-could-change-your-life-forever.html

Is Milk Gluten-Free? | BeyondCeliac.org. (n.d.). Beyond Celiac. https://www.beyondceliac.org/gluten-free-diet/is-it-gluten-free/milk/

It All Starts In Your Gut. (n.d.). BePure Wellness. Retrieved July 18, 2022, from https://bepure.co.nz/all-starts-in-gut#chapter1

Jacka, F. (2019). *What is the Gut Microbiome? – Food and Mood Centre*. Foodandmoodcentre.com.au. https://foodandmoodcentre.com.au/2016/07/what-is-the-gut-microbiome/

Jewell, T. (2017, September 19). *What Causes Dysbiosis and How Is It Treated?* Healthline. https://www.healthline.com/health/digestive-health/dysbiosis#outlook

Jimenez, F. L. (2021, June). *Caffeine: How does it affect blood pressure? - Mayo Clinic*. Www.mayoclinic.org. https://www.mayoclinic.org/diseases-conditions/high-blood-pressure/expert-answers/blood-pressure/FAQ-20058543?p=1

Joel. (2021, June 9). *Is Leaky Gut Real? - KnowYourDNA*. Know Your DNA. https://knowyourdna.com/is-leaky-gut-real/

Kinsinger, S. (2017, December). *Breathing Exercises to Improve Your Digestive Health | Blog*. Loyola Medicine. https://www.loyolamedicine.org/about-us/blog/how-breathing-exercises-relieve-stress-and-improve-digestive-health

Kubala, J. (2018, February 17). *Proteolytic Enzymes: How They Work, Benefits and Sources.* Healthline. https://www.healthline.com/nutrition/proteolytic-enzymes#TOC_TITLE_HDR_3

Lathrop, M. (n.d.). *Pesticides can ruin a health gut diet plan. Fruits and vegetables are tainted with pesticides, ruining stomach bacteria in your gut biome.* Ombre. Retrieved July 17, 2022, from https://www.ombrelab.com/blogs/immunity/pesticides-and-gi-problems

Leaky Gut and Dysbiosis | Beijing United Family Hospital and Clinics. (n.d.). Retrieved July 12, 2022, from https://beijing.ufh.com.cn/734/health-information/articles/leaky-gut-dysbiosis?lang=en

Leaky Gut Syndrome. (n.d.). Cleveland Clinic. https://my.clevelandclinic.org/health/diseases/22724-leaky-gut-syndrome

Li, W.-Z., Stirling, K., Yang, J.-J., & Zhang, L. (2020). Gut microbiota and diabetes: From correlation to causality and mechanism. *World Journal of Diabetes*, *11*(7), 293–308. https://doi.org/10.4239/wjd.v11.i7.293

Lobionda, S., Sittipo, P., Kwon, H. Y., & Lee, Y. K. (2019). The Role of Gut Microbiota in Intestinal Inflammation with Respect to Diet and Extrinsic Stressors. *Microorganisms*, *7*(8), 271. https://doi.org/10.3390/microorganisms7080271

MacGill, M. (2018, June 26). *Gut microbiota: Definition, importance, and medical uses.* Www.medicalnewstoday.com. https://www.medicalnewstoday.com/articles/307998#why-is-the-human-microbiota-important

Macmillan Cancer Support. (2020). *The oesophagus*. Macmillan.org.uk. https://www.macmillan.org.uk/cancer-information-and-support/oesophageal-cancer/the-oesophagus

Mandl, E. (2018, January 28). *The 7 Worst Foods for Your Brain*. Healthline. https://www.healthline.com/nutrition/worst-foods-for-your-brain#TOC_TITLE_HDR_2

Marasco, G., Di Biase, A. R., Schiumerini, R., Eusebi, L. H., Iughetti, L., Ravaioli, F., Scaioli, E., Colecchia, A., & Festi, D. (2016). Gut Microbiota and Celiac Disease. *Digestive Diseases and Sciences*, *61*(6), 1461–1472. https://doi.org/10.1007/s10620-015-4020-2

Mayo Clinic. (2018). *Irritable bowel syndrome - Symptoms and causes*. Mayo Clinic. https://www.mayoclinic.org/diseases-conditions/irritable-bowel-syndrome/symptoms-causes/syc-20360016

Mayo Clinic. (2020, October 14). *Water: How much should you drink every day?* Mayo Clinic. https://www.mayoclinic.org/healthy-lifestyle/nutrition-and-healthy-eating/in-depth/water/art-20044256

MayoClinic. (2016). *Don't get sabotaged by added sugar*. Mayo Clinic. https://www.mayoclinic.org/healthy-lifestyle/nutrition-and-healthy-eating/in-depth/added-sugar/art-20045328

McDonald, D., Hyde, E., Debelius, J. W., Morton, J. T., Gonzalez, A., Ackermann, G., Aksenov, A. A., Behsaz, B., Brennan, C., Chen, Y., DeRight Goldasich, L., Dorrestein, P. C., Dunn, R. R., Fahimipour, A. K., Gaffney, J., Gilbert, J. A., Gogul, G., Green, J. L., Hugenholtz, P., & Humphrey, G. (2018). American Gut: an Open Platform for Citizen Science Microbiome

Research. *MSystems*, *3*(3). https://doi.org/10.1128/msystems.00031-18

Mitsuhashi, S., Ballou, S., Jiang, Z. G., Hirsch, W., Nee, J., Iturrino, J., Cheng, V., & Lembo, A. (2018). Characterizing Normal Bowel Frequency and Consistency in a Representative Sample of Adults in the United States (NHANES). *American Journal of Gastroenterology*, *113*(1), 115–123. https://doi.org/10.1038/ajg.2017.213

Mulch, D. (2021, May 19). *7 Reasons Why The Burrito Bowl Is The Best Meal For Weight Loss*. In Fitness and in Health. https://medium.com/in-fitness-and-in-health/7-reasons-why-the-burrito-bowl-is-the-best-meal-for-weight-loss-84f7785abd02

Murakami, M., & Tognini, P. (2020). The Circadian Clock as an Essential Molecular Link Between Host Physiology and Microorganisms. *Frontiers in Cellular and Infection Microbiology*, *9*(Published online 2020 Jan 22. doi: 10.3389/fcimb.2019.00469). https://doi.org/10.3389/fcimb.2019.00469

Mutlu, E. A., Gillevet, P. M., Rangwala, H., Sikaroodi, M., Naqvi, A., Engen, P. A., Kwasny, M., Lau, C. K., & Keshavarzian, A. (2012). Colonic microbiome is altered in alcoholism. *American Journal of Physiology-Gastrointestinal and Liver Physiology*, *302*(9), G966–G978. https://doi.org/10.1152/ajpgi.00380.2011

Nasrallah, H. A. (2022, April). *Sexual activity alters the microbiome, with potential psychiatric implications*. Www.mdedge.com. https://www.mdedge.com/psychiatry/article/253221/mixed-topics/sexual-activity-alters-microbiome-potential-psychiatric

ND, C. G., Reboot Naturopath, B. HSc. (2015, April 11). *6 Great Benefits of Eating What's in Season*. Joe Cross. https://www.rebootwithjoe.com/benefits-of-eating-seasonally/#:~:text=Eating%20seasonally%20reduces%20the%20demand

Nielsen, L. N., Roager, H. M., Casas, M. E., Frandsen, H. L., Gosewinkel, U., Bester, K., Licht, T. R., Hendriksen, N. B., & Bahl, M. I. (2018). Glyphosate has limited short-term effects on commensal bacterial community composition in the gut environment due to sufficient aromatic amino acid levels. *Environmental Pollution, 233*(https://doi.org/10.1016/j.envpol.2017.10.016), 364–376. https://doi.org/10.1016/j.envpol.2017.10.016

Popov, S. (2021, May 21). *Free Gut Test You Can Do at Home | GUTXY*. GUTXY. https://www.gutxy.com/blog/free-gut-test-you-can-do-at-home/

Pot, J. (2022, April). *8 best journal apps of 2022 | Zapier*. Zapier.com. https://zapier.com/blog/best-journaling-apps/#penzu

published, T. L. (2014, April 25). *Poop Apps: 5 Tools for Tracking Your Stools*. Livescience.com. https://www.livescience.com/45150-apps-for-tracking-your-poop.html

Raman, R. (2017, July 2). *How to Do an Elimination Diet and Why*. Healthline. https://www.healthline.com/nutrition/elimination-diet#TOC_TITLE_HDR_4

Robertson, R. (2016, November 18). *10 Ways to Improve Your Gut Bacteria, Based on Science*. Healthline. https://www.healthline.com/nutrition/improve-gut-bacteria#TOC_TITLE_HDR_2

Robertson, R. (2017, July 25). *Why Bifidobacteria Are So Good for You.* Healthline. https://www.healthline.com/nutrition/why-bifidobacteria-are-good#TOC_TITLE_HDR_3

Robinson, L. (2020, October). *Mindful Eating - HelpGuide.org.* Https://Www.helpguide.org. https://www.helpguide.org/articles/diets/mindful-eating.htm

Sara. (2017, February 2). *Burrito Bowls with Chicken.* Dinner at the Zoo. https://www.dinneratthezoo.com/burrito-bowls-chicken/#recipe

Sender, R., Fuchs, S., & Milo, R. (2016). Revised Estimates for the Number of Human and Bacteria Cells in the Body. *PLOS Biology, 14*(8), e1002533. https://doi.org/10.1371/journal.pbio.1002533

Sirino, E. (2020, May 20). *Is Holding In Farts Healthy for You, Or Are There Side Effects?* Healthline. https://www.healthline.com/health/digestive-health/holding-in-farts#prevention

Small intestinal bacterial overgrowth (SIBO) - Symptoms and causes. (n.d.). Mayo Clinic. https://www.mayoclinic.org/diseases-conditions/small-intestinal-bacterial-overgrowth/symptoms-causes/syc-20370168

Stomach Secretion - an overview | ScienceDirect Topics. (n.d.). Www.sciencedirect.com. https://www.sciencedirect.com/topics/medicine-and-dentistry/stomach-secretion

Strait, L. (2022, May 4). *The 9 Healthiest Beans and Legumes You Can Eat.* Healthline.

https://www.healthline.com/nutrition/healthiest-beans-legumes#soybeans

Suez, J., Korem, T., Zeevi, D., Zilberman-Schapira, G., Thaiss, C. A., Maza, O., Israeli, D., Zmora, N., Gilad, S., Weinberger, A., Kuperman, Y., Harmelin, A., Kolodkin-Gal, I., Shapiro, H., Halpern, Z., Segal, E., & Elinav, E. (2014). Artificial sweeteners induce glucose intolerance by altering the gut microbiota. *Nature*, *514*(7521), 181–186. https://doi.org/10.1038/nature13793

The central role of the gut. (2022). Danone Nutricia Research. https://www.nutriciaresearch.com/gut-and-microbiology/the-central-role-of-the-gut/

The Digestive System. (n.d.). Love Your Gut. Retrieved July 3, 2022, from https://loveyourgut.com/what-does-the-gut-do/the-digestive-system/

The Elimination Diet. (2018). https://www.fammed.wisc.edu/files/webfm-uploads/documents/outreach/im/handout_elimination_diet_patient.pdf

The Ins and Outs. (n.d.). Love Your Gut. Retrieved July 3, 2022, from https://loveyourgut.com/what-does-the-gut-do/the-ins-and-outs/

Tooley, K. L. (2020). Effects of the Human Gut Microbiota on Cognitive Performance, Brain Structure and Function: A Narrative Review. *Nutrients*, *12*(10), 3009. https://doi.org/10.3390/nu12103009

Underwood, E. (2018, September 20). *Your gut is directly connected to your brain, by a newly discovered neuron circuit.* Www.science.org. https://www.science.org/content/article/your-gut-directly-connected-your-brain-newly-discovered-neuron-circuit

Vijay, A., & Valdes, A. M. (2021). Role of the gut microbiome in chronic diseases: a narrative review. *European Journal of Clinical Nutrition, Published online 2021 Sep 28. doi: 10.1038/s41430-021-00991-6*, 1–13. https://doi.org/10.1038/s41430-021-00991-6

Viome Team. (2018, June 13). *Why is Celiac Disease on the Rise?* Viome.com. https://www.viome.com/blog/why-celiac-disease-rise-answer-gut-microbiome

Virieze, J. D. (2014, March 12). *Crohn's Disease Marked by Dramatic Changes in Gut Bacteria.* Www.science.org. https://www.science.org/content/article/crohns-disease-marked-dramatic-changes-gut-bacteria

Water Science School. (2019, May 22). *The Water in You: Water and the Human Body | U.S. Geological Survey.* Www.usgs.gov. https://www.usgs.gov/special-topics/water-science-school/science/water-you-water-and-human-body

What Are Emulsifiers, and What Do They Do in Our Food? (2021, May 7). Food Insight. https://foodinsight.org/emulsifiers-in-food/

What Is Your Gut Telling You? (n.d.). Love Your Gut. Retrieved July 19, 2022, from https://loveyourgut.com/what-does-the-gut-do/what-is-your-gut-telling-you/

What You Need to Know About Coffee. (n.d.). BePure Wellness. Retrieved July 23, 2022, from https://bepure.co.nz/what-need-know-about-coffee?_pos=1&_sid=d5f742a4f&_ss=r

Wu, Y., Xu, J., Rong, X., Wang, F., Wang, H., & Zhao, C. (2021). Gut microbiota alterations and health status in aging adults: From correlation to causation. *AGING MEDICINE*, *4*(3), 206–213. https://doi.org/10.1002/agm2.12167

Xu, M., Qi, Q., Liang, J., Bray, G. A., Hu, F. B., Sacks, F. M., & Qi, L. (2013). Genetic Determinant for Amino Acid Metabolites and Changes in Body Weight and Insulin Resistance in Response to Weight-Loss Diets. *Circulation*, *127*(12), 1283–1289. https://doi.org/10.1161/circulationaha.112.000586

Young, C. (2019). *What is the Gut Microbiome? – Food and Mood Centre*. Foodandmoodcentre.com.au. https://foodandmoodcentre.com.au/2016/07/what-is-the-gut-microbiome/

Zinc deficiency reduces digestive enzymes. (2019, July 16). Www.scientificwellness.com. https://www.scientificwellness.com/blog-view/zinc-deficiency-reduces-digestive-enzymes-548

Printed in Great Britain
by Amazon